Teaching and Learning in Clinical Settings

Richard Hays
Professor of Medical Education
Keele University

Forewords by

Dame Lesley Southgate
Professor of Medical Education
St George's University of London

and

Elisabeth Paice
Director, London Deanery

Radcliffe Publishing
Oxford • Seattle

Radcliffe Publishing Ltd
18 Marcham Road
Abingdon
Oxon OX14 1AA
United Kingdom

www.radcliffe-oxford.com
Electronic catalogue and worldwide online ordering facility.

British Library Cataloguing in Publication Data

A catalogue record for this book is available from the British Library.

ISBN-10 1 85775 751 3
ISBN-13 978 1 85775 751 4

Typeset by Anne Joshua & Associates, Oxford
Printed and bound by TJ International Ltd, Padstow, Cornwall

Contents

Foreword

Teaching and learning in any clinical setting is difficult to plan, absolutely dependent on the context, and frequently has to compete with service commitments for the time and attention of teachers and learners alike. But removal of learners to the classroom or lecture theatre, or even to small group work isolated from clinical care, leads to a dislocation of theory from practice that may be difficult to recover from in the undergraduate years.

The development of expertise is related to experience in the expert's area of practice. And its foundations lie in the clinical encounters in medical school, often remembered with great clarity many years later. This learning from patients is enhanced by exposure to effective role models who demonstrate professionalism and reinforce the student's motivation to succeed.

But unplanned clinical teaching which is not referenced to an explicit curriculum to which the assessment programme is mapped, can lead to perverse outcomes. Students need time to reflect on what they are learning, and to make sense of the snapshots of patients' lives that they are privileged to see. This is especially true of the patients that may be seen once or twice in hospital, while very ill, where the focus of the student's attention may be on the diagnosis and management of the disease and the buzz of saving a life. It takes excellent clinical teaching to remember to explore how the situation might have been prevented, or the difficulties of the recovery phase or long-term follow up. And to highlight the roles of other health professionals in care.

This book explores all of these issues from a practical standpoint illustrated with many examples. The reader is also offered the theoretical basis for planning and delivering clinical teaching in a way that enables the teacher to use opportunities, maximise chances and to develop an environment where effective learning coexists with the pressures and other priorities of busy clinical care.

Dame Lesley Southgate
Professor of Medical Education
St George's University of London
November 2005

Foreword

Nothing drives adult learning like a practical demonstration of the 'need to know' in a real-life setting. Richard Hays well understands how much of the added value of the clinical setting for teaching is in helping learners visualise their future role as the practitioner, and develop that passionate 'need to know' which will drive their learning long after exams are a dim memory. His book on teaching and learning in clinical settings reflects his extensive experience of facilitating this process. He takes the same approach to educating the teachers and trainers. This book abounds in realistic recognisable scenarios that help the reader visualise the situation described, empathise with the participants, and reflect on the lessons contained within it. Having read three or four of these scenarios, the reader is well-primed with the 'need to know' and well-motivated to take in the excellent advice contained toward the end of each chapter and summarised in boxes of key points. All is written in a lucid prose devoid of educational jargon. This is a gem of a book that anyone engaged in clinical teaching will learn from and will enjoy reading.

Professor Elisabeth Paice
Director, London Deanery
November 2005

Preface

This book was written because of the success, and failure, of a book I wrote to guide general practitioners to become better clinical supervisors. That book combined a practical approach to teaching and learning with some education theory to help busy clinicians gain a deeper understanding of their teaching roles and develop as teachers. The book has been surprisingly successful with primary care clinical teachers, but one of its probable strengths for that context – its connection to primary care – has not made the education messages as accessible to clinical teachers in other medical disciplines. Even though the educational messages are the same, hospital-based clinicians have to teach in a different context, with somewhat different pressures. My experience as Dean of a new medical school has shown me that that is the group – hospital-based clinicians – that most needs access to professional development resources in medical education, because medical education is expanding rapidly. More students are in the healthcare system, more hospitals are taking students, postgraduate education is becoming more formal (e.g. the Foundation Years), and more clinicians are being asked to take on teaching and supervision roles.

Hence this book has been written for a more general audience, but with particular relevance to inpatient and other large clinical settings. The formula is similar, in that there is a combination of the practical and the theory that underpins practice, but there is greater emphasis on scenarios that provide glimpses of teaching and learning practices. The scenarios are all based on real situations I have experienced or observed as either a learner, a teacher or a manager of teaching. They are arranged before the more theoretical material, as perhaps they demonstrate the theory better than reading theory. There is more than enough theory for some, perhaps enough for those wanting to take on substantive teaching roles, and perhaps not enough for those wanting to become leaders of teaching programmes. However, each chapter includes a brief annotated bibliography of mostly recent reviews or primary research in medical education, so those who want to pursue greater knowledge have somewhere to start.

Richard Hays
November 2005

About the author

Richard Hays went into full-time rural procedural and then general practice for a few years before being asked to help teach GP registrars and medical students. He soon realised how little he knew about medical education, and then embarked on a career in academic medicine. He has both a PhD in education and an MD in medical education, and he has worked for 20 years in both postgraduate and undergraduate medical education, including establishing a new medical school at James Cook University in Australia. He maintains part-time clinical practice as well as teaching in both community and hospital settings. He has written several book chapters and books on rural health and medical education, and has published about 100 research papers. From early 2006 he is the Head of the new medical school at Keele University in the United Kingdom.

Part 1

The context of clinical teaching

Chapter 1

Developing as a learner and a teacher

Competent clinicians provide patient care.
Incompetent clinicians teach.
Incompetent teachers become managers.
Incompetent managers get promoted.

Anon

Introduction

Medical students should learn from more experienced people within their chosen profession, as well as related professions, in a range of clinical settings that reflect current professional practice. Therefore, medical schools need to recruit and support a large number of clinicians who are willing and able to facilitate this learning. Many clinicians accept a teaching role because they acknowledge a professional obligation, but do not have the time or interest to explore in great depth the whys and wherefores. They are interested in contributing to student learning, but not many will have received any formal instruction in how to do this well. This chapter discusses how competent clinicians can also become competent teachers and presents a brief introduction to some important teaching and learning concepts, at the same time exposing some of the common myths that pervade clinical teaching.

Levels of involvement with clinical teaching

Clinical teachers are usually clinicians first and teachers second. This reflects the nature of their work, as the teaching role is usually part of a primarily clinical service role in a health facility, and they may not be paid explicitly for their teaching role. Hence most clinical teachers would regard their teaching role as a part-time involvement in the practical side of medical education. Fortunately, the profession of medicine values the teaching role highly and most clinicians are willing to contribute.

The simplest and most common involvement is where a clinician agrees to supervise a student, or a group of students, in the clinical setting. Many are also asked to contribute to case discussions or provide a tutorial for small groups of students, generally within the healthcare facility. A smaller number may be asked to give a lecture or contribute to a seminar for larger groups, perhaps the whole year cohort. Almost all will be asked to contribute to the assessment of students, particularly the clinical assessment. Some will be invited to join curriculum planning or management committees within the medical school. This book aims to help clinicians develop in all of these roles.

Myth #1. All experienced clinicians are good teachers.

Clinical expertise and teaching expertise

It is almost certainly true that one of the requirements of clinical teachers is that they are sound, competent clinicians. Teachers need to have content knowledge and skills relevant to their discipline. However, content knowledge and skills are not the only determinants of competence; competent clinicians cannot know everything, and they are aware of their limitations and know where to find current information. So long as clinical teachers do not pretend that they know everything, they can be effective facilitators of learning. An extension of this is the assumption that only a specialist can teach medical students about the particular specialty. For example, should all medical students be taught how to examine the abdomen by a gastroenterologist or a colorectal surgeon? If only we had enough of them to do that, says the course coordinator! The obvious answer is no. Generalists, either general practitioners or 'generalist specialists', are often the best teachers of basic skills because they are aware of the many purposes for basic history taking and examination skills, and the many directions such a patient encounter may go. Certainly, at the postgraduate specialty training level, trainee specialists need to be taught the more subtle skills necessary for practising that specialty, but that level of expertise is less important at medical student level. Another advantage of the generalists is that they are more numerous and available.

A commonly made assumption is that all experienced clinicians will be good teachers. However appealing this notion is, the reality is that the correlation between clinical expertise and educational expertise is not good. These are two different sets of skills, so why should they be correlated? The academic roles of teaching, assessing and managing each require skills that clinicians are not usually taught as part of their own clinical training. These skills can be acquired by clinicians, some more easily than others. Putting to one side the different skills required for committee membership, as these are beyond the scope of this book, the most difficult sets of skills to acquire are probably those required for managing small groups, supervising students and assessing students. This does not mean that giving a guest lecture to a large group is necessarily easy, but it is at least a familiar, respected and better recognised format. Speaking in a large darkened room to a personal collection of exotic images and acquired wisdom, with a few questions at the end, is quite different to dealing with small groups of or individual learners on different, patient-generated agendas, because of different capacities to track the learning progress of individual students. In lectures, this is rarely achievable, whereas in smaller groups, it is not only achievable, but mandatory. Sadly, most clinical teachers find themselves supervising small groups of students without any preparation or professional educational development, and with little understanding of the curriculum and assessment processes of newer integrated courses.

It is not that experienced clinicians cannot be good teachers, but more that quite inexperienced clinicians can also be very good teachers, and that clinicians at all levels can be poor teachers. Learners often learn a lot from colleagues just a short distance ahead of them, so junior medical students can learn a lot from senior students, as do senior students from junior resident medical officers and registrars. People just ahead often know the curriculum and the practical side of implementing it better than more senior clinicians. Effective teaching is more about communication and connection with learners than with individual content brilliance or experience.

Hence this book is aimed quite deliberately at more junior clinicians as well as the more experienced people now seeking a broader professional role.

> **Myth #2. All I have to demonstrate is sound clinical knowledge and skills.**

More than just clinical teaching and learning

While clinical teachers are employed to help students learn clinical knowledge and skills, it is no longer sufficient to just have technical expertise in individual patient care. One of the more current issues facing clinical teachers is that a curriculum now expects students to gain more from their clinical placements than mere clinical knowledge and skills. Although clinical care of individual patients is still the biggest part of medical practice, we increasingly have to take a population approach to tackling health problems in a range of primary and secondary care settings. Further, society expects doctors to be honest, reliable, diligent, accountable and able to remain current in their knowledge and skills. Finally, the profession, particularly the younger members, expects doctors to have more balanced lives, able to be partners, parents and community members as well as clinicians. These aspects are formally included in curriculum themes or 'domains', and should be demonstrated by clinical teachers. Clinical teachers should be seen to be well balanced in their personal and professional lives, to have both the desire and the ability to maintain currency and practise evidence-based medicine, and to understand both the whole patient and the patient's environment.

This perhaps presents an almost superhuman position description, and medical schools will settle for much less, so long as clinical teachers are aware of their limits and seek advice on their teaching role, just as they all would for the clinical role.

> **Myth #3. All researchers are good clinical teachers.**

Research expertise and teaching expertise

It is often the case that the more academic clinicians are assumed to automatically be good clinical teachers. These individuals are often up with the latest information and may be making a personal contribution to the advancement of knowledge through their own clinical research. One of the common truisms in higher education is that teaching and research are complementary, each informing the other.

But are they necessarily good teachers? The answer, of course, is no. Research and teaching are both academic activities, but require different sets of skills. Many researchers tend to be a little introverted, rather serious about their interests (even changing lectures to their own research), inclined to overly theoretical explanations, and quite sceptical. Some are not wonderful at interpersonal communication. Researchers are often better at postgraduate research supervision than undergraduate teaching.

Before researchers reading this book rip it up and withdraw from teaching, let me say quickly that researchers can be very good teachers and role models, but they might need to acquire the different set of skills, if they do not already possess it.

Myth #4. Attendance at teaching courses produces expert clinical teachers.

Developing as a teacher

The first thing that prospective clinical teachers must ask of themselves is 'do I want to teach?' Hippocratic philosophy suggests that all medical practitioners should help prepare the next generation of doctors, and this principle is becoming enshrined in formal role descriptions of medical practitioners, but clinical medicine and teaching require different sets of knowledge and skills and not all of us can be good at both. If the answer to the question is no, then good clinicians should get on with being good clinicians. There are of course other ways to facilitate learning, such as supporting others in the healthcare team to teach while the clinical work is done.

If the answer to the question is yes, then clinicians should explore why they want to teach. Motivation to teach is very important as there are few extrinsic rewards for clinical teachers. Healthcare facilities are geared to provide efficient, high-quality healthcare, and learners do not necessarily fit easily into that environment. Being a good teacher is not usually rewarded in employment conditions, and although universities may offer a few trimmings such as academic titles, library cards and guidance with research, teaching often adds to the working hours of already busy people. This is not much of a problem for clinicians who *want* to teach and *enjoy* teaching, as that is the intrinsic reward. Some teaching hospitals are sufficiently imbued with the academic culture for teaching to be formally required and supported, but this is not the norm in many healthcare facilities.

If this thinking reveals a motivated teacher, then each person should explore his or her ability to teach. Teaching skills are not innate, although personality factors are important. Learners can learn from many kinds of clinicians, even the poor teachers, although they can learn the wrong things! Box 1.1 lists some of the desirable attributes in teachers found in education research. These include a combination of knowledge, skills and attitudes, some of which are not easy to learn. Perhaps it is easier to think of the opposite to these attributes, as they have been shown to be present in ineffective teachers being autocratic, aloof, dull, boring, evasive and erratic.

An important question then looms. How can sound clinicians acquire these attributes and become sound teachers? The obvious answer is to attend a course in clinical teaching. However, while that is almost certainly a useful activity, clinicians who have not made it to step one – motivation to teach and learn how to improve – will probably not gain much from attendance. Just as attendance at continuing medical education (CME) events is a weak measure of continuing professional development, attendance at teacher training sessions is insufficient to guarantee that attendees will develop as teachers. In addition, attendees need to reflect on their teaching practices, seek feedback on their performance, learn from each other and perhaps read some education theory to better understand what they must do.

Box 1.1 Desirable attributes in clinical teachers

- Motivated to help learners learn.
- Effective communication skills.
- Understanding of students' needs.
- Aware of own expertise as both clinician and teacher.
- Respectful of learners.
- Fair and democratic in dealings with learners.
- Responsive to needs of learners.
- Original and entertaining.
- Alert and confident.

Myth #5. Students are all bright so it does not matter what I do as a teacher.

Understanding students' needs

Clinicians have all been students and have been (still are?) recipients of an enormous amount of medical education. Although this experience does not guarantee that clinicians are good teachers, it can influence the way in which they approach their teaching role.

Their experience will often suggest that they learned almost despite the surrounding health and education system. Medical students tend to be high academic achievers who develop interests and have the energy and the ability to learn a combination of what they need to learn and what they want to learn. Most clinical teachers have successfully negotiated this process and may even have done well. They will remember the variable educational experiences that they and their peers had, and may well assume that their contribution to current medical students may well not make much difference to their outcomes, reflecting a touch of cynicism.

The truth is closer to the opposite of this myth. Students will learn the curriculum on their own if they have to, as learners will do what it takes to pass an examination. However, they will achieve more efficiently and appropriately if they are guided through the curriculum by teachers who know the path and can nudge learners back on track if they stray too far. This does not mean spoon feeding. Research indicates that the largest source of error variance in teaching quality is often the teachers.

Myth #6. This worked for me so it will work for them.

Further, many clinicians will base their teaching style on their own medical student experiences of clinical teachers. These can be strong influences, even where the experience is not remembered as particularly positive. Sometimes being a stern critic is regarded as being necessary. The 'rites of passage' concept often appears, at least sub-minimally – 'I survived and am now a competent practitioner, so the techniques I experienced must be OK for everyone else too'.

Neither of these approaches is helpful to medical students, who are, more than ever, confronted with a potentially huge curriculum and a long period in which to achieve their ultimate career goal. Current medical students are usually in different kinds of curricula to those experienced by most current clinicians. These days problem-based learning (PBL) and other forms of integrated, more interactive curricula are widespread. Students are used to framing questions, even challenging orthodoxy, and seeking resources to answer their questions. They are more used to having their opinions respected.

Sound clinical teachers get to understand the needs of both the group of students, and of the individuals within their group, and try to make learning a positive experience. Negative learning experiences can profoundly affect what and how students learn and successful learning should not be left to chance.

Clinical teachers should instead focus on their memories of their more positive or inspirational learning interactions with past clinical teachers. It is likely that most will relate to powerful, positive role modelling by clinicians who were exemplary clinicians, teachers and human beings, people who appeared to care and who took time and energy to help learners learn. Such people do not necessarily have to have a great knowledge of education theory, nor even necessarily be great teachers of clinical material, because they just stand out from the rest and inspire others to emulate them. Many clinicians chose their postgraduate careers because of interaction with such a person. This is the power of role modelling, one of the least understood yet most powerful influences in personal development

The continuum of expertise

This then shapes both the first, and to some extent the highest, levels of attributes required of clinical teachers. At a minimum, clinical teachers should be motivated to help others learn. They should also be aware of their own learning experiences, in particular what worked well for their personal learning style. They should try to emulate the more positive experiences and be wary of the more negative. Ideally, all clinical teachers at this early stage will attend teacher development programmes conducted by their medical school.

At the highest level we will find those eminent, awe-inspiring clinical teachers who seem to be experts at motivating people to learn, as well as being expert at helping them learn. Many of these great teachers will not be conscious of why and how they do such a good job, as they just may have the right combination of intuition and experience, without any theoretical understanding. Between these extremes of the spectrum are people with increasing levels of expertise in helping people learn, based on their knowledge and skills of the educational attributes discussed below. Some may develop just on intuition and experience, but a bit of understanding and training should aid that development.

One set of attributes that should be developed to improve as a clinical teacher includes knowledge of how people learn (there are different learning styles), how to assess performance, and how to give constructive feedback. These are the basic tools of the education process. They are not hard to learn and they are presented briefly in later chapters of this book.

Another set of attributes necessary to improve as a clinical teacher relates to achieving a deep understanding of one's own level of expertise as a teacher and learner and how this impacts on helping others to learn. This requires some feedback from others and, ideally, some self-evaluation of teaching performance. Universities can usually provide student feedback for clinical teachers, although their systems are better for more permanent staff than for part-time teaching by external clinical teaching staff, most of whom are not formally employed by universities. Medical schools should be able to arrange for more individual teaching evaluations. If not, the information provided in Chapter 6 should be helpful to those wanting to organise teaching evaluations. If done well (de-identified, involving several groups over several terms, collected and analysed by an independent person), such evaluations can provide meaningful feedback to clinical teachers and guide further development.

Self-evaluation is a powerful method of obtaining feedback. Here, clinical teachers can listen to audiotapes or observe videotapes of their encounters with students. Again, medical schools should be able to assist with this, but a self-evaluation instrument is provided in Chapter 6 for those who want to do this independently. Beware that self-observation can be very challenging, as we often focus on our voice and mannerisms more than the educational substance, and sometimes do not like what we hear and see! Try to get beyond that. Sharing a video with a trusted colleague is often helpful, and sharing it with a respected and more experienced educator may offer insights benchmarked against other clinical teachers. Achieving this kind of understanding of teaching and learning processes can lead to the development of very high achievement as a clinical teacher.

Myth #7. Using new technology makes teaching more effective.

Technical wizardry

Teaching institutions are full of modern technology. It is now possible to have slide presentations with not just clear colour images, but video clips and additional sound and visual effects, such as individualised colours, backgrounds and slide transitions. Preparing a presentation can be a lot of fun, particularly for the technically minded, and can add interest by presenting information in interesting ways. Teaching around patients can utilise hand-held personal computers (PCs) with wireless connections to the internet, so that the latest evidence can be sought to support decision making, drug interactions can be checked, and contributions can be made to the patient record, all at the bedside.

However appealing it is to think that using new electronic and communications technology makes teaching more effective, this is not necessarily the case. Indeed, the opposite effect may well be seen if technology is not used well.

Special effects should be used sparingly in slide presentations so that they do not distract learners from their main task. Like a good cartoon, special effects can grab attention, relieve tension or indicate change of topics, but when overdone can diminish the message and perhaps even drive the audience crazy.

Using hand-held PCs also has limits, partly because they are less useful without substantial technical support (wireless connections, interactive software and information technology [IT] technicians), and partly because the technology, rather than the patients, can become the focus of the learning task.

While clinical teachers should use current technology in their teaching, they should consider the almost timeless debate: should technology drive the development of educational methods, or the reverse? In reality both processes occur, but teachers should probably avoid using technology unless there is either a strong rationale (ideally with research evidence) or at least a reasonable expectation of some benefit. Further, teachers need to master the technology before applying it, and should do so sparingly until benefits are obvious.

Myth #8. All clinical teachers should obtain educational qualifications.

Educational qualifications

The move to formalise and professionalise clinical teaching inevitably leads to the question: should clinical teachers obtain formal educational qualifications?

The answer, as for so many questions about life, is: it all depends!

To begin with, formal qualifications do not convert a poor teacher into a good teacher and many excellent clinical teachers do not have formal educational qualifications. These rules of thumb will probably always be true.

A desire to obtain formal qualifications is probably a personal decision, based on both intrinsic and extrinsic factors. Extrinsic factors include rewards provided by the system, such as assistance with promotion, additional allowances or additional privileges. For clinicians employed in the broader healthcare system, there are few extrinsic rewards, as seniority is usually based on professional and clinical criteria, such as clinical experience, but other criteria might become important in the future, so clinicians aiming for advancement may not be wasting time seeking formal educational qualifications. Such qualifications would assist in gaining higher-level clinical or academic titles within medical schools.

The most important rewards are almost certainly intrinsic, as this is just doing something for the satisfaction of achieving a personal goal. Clinicians interested in teaching and learning are likely to enjoy learning how they can do this well. It is likely that those who are interested may already be good teachers, so intrinsic rewards may not help the less motivated and less able.

Should a clinical teacher want to gain some formal educational qualification, the next question is: what is available?

The answer, sadly, is not much. Many universities run Graduate Certificates of Teaching (or similar nomenclature), but these are often more about the more structured large group activities commonly employed in universities – lectures, seminars, etc. – rather than the small group and one-to-one processes more often employed in medical education. These are usually quite practical, but the content varies and some shopping around is worthwhile to select the right subjects and courses.

Those with a more academic interest might benefit from a Masters-level programme that includes a lot more theory. These are being established in most nations, so check the websites of local medical schools. Two of the best known international programmes are available from the University of Dundee (www.dundee.ac.uk) in Scotland and the University of Maastricht (www. unimaas.nl) in the Netherlands. Both are available using both flexible delivery and some residential attendance.

For the really serious clinical educators, it is possible to construct a more self-directed, but much more ambitious, learning pathway through conducting formal, supervised medical education research leading to a Professional Doctorate or a PhD. This requires three years' full-time or six to eight years' part-time enrolment, and a strong will to see it through despite conflicting demands on a very busy life. Those choosing this path will probably end up in educational research or management roles. A more recent and perhaps more manageable path is that of the Professional Doctorate in Medical Education. The format varies, but involves the development of a portfolio for submission, like a PhD thesis, but including the products of several more 'bite-sized' educational development and research tasks.

> **Myth #9. There are few rewards for clinicians who devote time to teaching.**

Recognising and rewarding clinical teaching

Extrinsic rewards for part-time clinical teaching are often not obvious. Most clinical teachers have full-time clinical roles where patient care generally takes first priority, even when employment contracts include time allocated for academic activities. A lot depends on the nature of the local healthcare system and the way in which budgets are resourced. Universities often do make contributions to hospital systems to 'buy' protected time from clinicians, but these arrangements can be difficult to unravel. Regardless of the nature of employment contracts, if clinicians are overloaded with clinical work, they feel as if their teaching is in 'free' time.

Arguably the most transparent system is where universities directly employ clinical teachers in addition to their health system responsibilities, but this is not always possible. Further, teaching is usually less well remunerated than clinical work, so 'full' payment for teaching services is rarely possible.

Medical schools should take this issue seriously and negotiate appropriate arrangements with their clinical teachers, who are the mainstay of teaching in senior years of medical programmes. Some extrinsic rewards are not difficult to achieve. Examples include academic titles, limited support for research (facilities and methodology advice), access to university libraries and access to professional development opportunities. These cost the university very little and can mean a lot.

Hence intrinsic rewards remain the most available and important in most healthcare systems. Luckily, they are abundant and free. Most student contact is positive, as students generally want to learn and clinicians generally want to teach. This is the main source of satisfaction for clinical teachers. Student interactions can be enjoyable, they provoke clinicians to keep up to date, and clinical teachers enjoy seeing 'their' students go on to do interesting things, even if not in their own specialty. Most clinicians are happy to offer their services without a lot of thought about genuine rewards. Clinicians who do not enjoy teaching probably should not do it, as lack of intrinsic rewards may not provide adequate compensation for the effort.

How to use this book

This book should be regarded as a primer for clinical teachers, aimed at those at all levels of the professional teaching development spectrum. It is divided into three parts. Part 1 provides current information about being a clinical teacher. Part 2 includes the practical chapters that deal with the 'how to' of clinical teaching in the current healthcare context. Part 3 provides some theoretical background to curriculum development, assessment and evaluation. While this order has a certain logic, the three parts can be read in any order. More experiential learners will prefer to start with the more practical, experiential chapters (3–5) before encountering the theory. These chapters use scenarios extensively to illustrate important issues and prime interest in theory. This is similar to the approach of most modern medical curricula, including PBL curricula. Others may prefer to start with the more theoretical chapters (6–8), absorbing and understanding the theory before applying it to the scenarios.

Where possible, the discussion is based on educational evidence. Each chapter includes a recommended further reading list for those who wish to delve more deeply into the issues. The resources are annotated, focusing more on the most relevant and most commonly available resources. A list of references (books, journals and websites) is provided to guide those wanting a more academic experience of the available evidence. Finally, the book concludes with a glossary of medical education terms that clinical teachers will encounter in curriculum documents and discussions.

Summary

This first chapter has really just set the scene for those readers who want to improve their skills in helping learners learn in clinical settings, and has described current thinking about models of clinical teaching. The next chapter provides an overview of some current issues in clinical teaching, prior to a more practical, scenario-based exploration of teaching and assessment skills.

Further reading

- Busari JO, Weggelaar NM, Knottnerus AC *et al.* (2005) How medical residents perceive the quality of supervision provided by attending doctors in the clinical setting. *Medical Education.* **39**: 696–705.
  Research reporting student views on what works best for them.
- Cottrell D, Kilminster S, Jolly B *et al.* (2002) What is effective supervision and how does it happen? A critical incident study. *Medical Education.* **36**: 1042–9.
  Research that shows that learners and teachers sometimes have differing views on the best way to teach and learn.
- Markert RJ (2001) What makes a good teacher? Lessons from teaching medical students. *Academic Medicine.* **76**: 809–10.
  Wise words from an experienced teacher.

Chapter 2

An overview of clinical teaching issues

Neither talent without instruction, nor instruction without talent, can produce the perfect craftsman.

Vitruvius, *c*.25 BC

Introduction

Without clinical teaching, medical students would not be able to place their theoretical learning in a practical context and would require a lot more support at internship and junior house officer (JHO) level to be safe to release on the public. At least that is the assertion that is accepted by nearly everybody in medical education, but there is not much research evidence, probably because most regard it as an obvious truism and have not done any such research.

However, the nature of clinical teaching has changed over time, not so much because of the nature of the education process required, but because of the profound changes in the healthcare system and the development of formal career pathways that require a university education at the first step. This chapter provides a brief overview of the history of the development of clinical teaching and then discusses some current topics that must be faced by clinical teachers.

The origins of clinical teaching

Clinical placements are the mainstay of medical education. The more recent tradition of having defined clinical rotations, terms or placements in hospital settings gained wider prominence as a result of the Flexner Report in 1911 in the USA, as the author recommended that medical schools adopt a pre-clinical science and clinical attachment structure, the latter consisting of small group or individual attachments to experienced clinicians, mostly in teaching hospitals. The Flexner Report was actually more concerned with the role of pre-clinical science in medical curricula, and the clinical attachment period was very similar in concept to the traditional 'practicum' that medical schools had introduced some centuries before, and really not much different to the apprenticeship model that we hear so much about, except that that was usually a one-to-one experience with a mentor.

Since the advent of teaching hospitals in Europe around a thousand years ago, houses of healing that were open to the public have been used as places for medical students to learn. Here there was a steady supply of usually very sick people, mostly with infectious diseases or conditions that might respond to the rather crude surgical processes of the time, and with few choices in healthcare. Death rates were high as there were few treatments and surgery was, until the advent of safe anaesthesia, a very risky business. The hospitals were charitable organisations, often Church run, that provided a caring environment. Doctors usually worked predominantly in private practice, donating their time (hence the term 'honorary') to hospitals for more interesting medicine and to teach.

Over the centuries the more recent model of a teaching hospital evolved. Typically, a city would have one or several large teaching hospitals with concentrated facilities and staff providing a wide range of clinical services to patients in surrounding suburbs. Nursing and medical students were part of the fabric, the former usually working, the latter usually visiting with the doctors. Large numbers of patients with a wide range of conditions often stayed many days for investigations, treatments and recovery. Medical students had many opportunities to learn from patients, through both formal and informal processes. The formal processes included the honorary doctor's ward rounds, where students could observe in detail the healthcare episodes of several patients; in time formal meetings also developed, such as grand rounds, death review meetings, etc. The informal learning involved seeing patients in the wards. By the 1970s, when I was a medical student, there were registrars and JHOs to learn from, each on a different career pathway level, but learning from each other and teaching those on lower levels.

By early in the twenty-first century, however, teaching hospitals have changed substantially. They are now smaller, with fewer beds, but much busier and more *efficient* at dealing with patients (bed numbers are no longer an accurate guide to hospital activity). They contain some amazing, and amazingly expensive, technology and technologists, and provide powerful new methods of diagnosis and treatment. The experience of patients is also very different, as many more (now up to 50% of the total) attend on a same-day basis, or at least for very short stays, as investigations and post-operative care become more ambulatory or home-based. Many of the longer-term staying patients are so sick, or have such complex medical problems, that medical students may not interact with them at all. Post-admission ward rounds have become essentially service-focused. Many hospitals are so busy providing clinical care that finding time to teach is becoming increasingly difficult.

The professional environment has also changed. Funders expect graduates to be able to meet the needs of the population (hence greater focus on mental health and aged care). The public now expects medical practice to be safe, with few errors and, when errors do occur, an identified cause. Greater emphasis is now placed on improving accountability in an era of increasing medical litigation and increasing difficulties with professional indemnity. Medical students are increasingly judged as junior members of the profession, with some of the responsibilities and accountabilities of the profession. Personal and professional development issues are now much more prominent.

Hence the approach to curriculum and assessment design has had to change. It is no longer possible to provide students with sufficient knowledge and skills to be a competent, independent practitioner beyond a basic level. Medical knowledge is developing rapidly, and all of it cannot possibly be taught. If new material is added, it has to be at the expense of something that is removed. Most programmes have less of the basic sciences than 20 years ago and can only provide sufficient clinical science to enable graduates to commence internship. Hence curriculum reform is universal and almost constant. Concepts such as integration, problem-based and resource-based learning and early clinical exposure are now commonly discussed and implemented. A major focus is on equipping students to constantly update knowledge and skills throughout a long career, rather than on 'information overload'. Most medical schools now have medical education units to provide the in-house expertise to support curriculum and assessment practices.

A final pressure is that in many parts of the world medical schools are expanding and new ones are being established to provide the workforce that is needed for an increasing and ageing population. As a result, teaching facilities are becoming rather overcrowded, with the potential to dilute clinical experience further. One could wonder about the accuracy of many workforce reports, as recent graduates appear to work differently from previous generations, and career options and pathways are changing, but we have to find a way of training more *efficiently*. The increasing use of skills labs, simulated patients and computer simulations are in part an attempt for this greater efficiency.

These changes have resulted in profound changes to the way medical schools approach their task. Current trends in medical school education are summarised in Box 2.1.

One outcome of these trends is that being a part-time teacher in a teaching facility is probably not as simple as it used to be. All clinical teachers probably need to know a bit about the curriculum and assessment processes experienced by their students.

Box 2.1 Summary of current trends in medical school education

- Medical school curricula no longer even try to provide all possible relevant knowledge in basic and clinical sciences.
- Hospital experiences should be augmented by primary care and community experiences to provide sufficient breadth of exposure to curriculum content.
- Professional and ethical issues have become more prominent as medical schools aim to produce graduates with particular behaviours and attitudes in addition to knowledge and skills.
- Patient simulations are being used more often, both for patient safety and to cope with the mismatch between student numbers and available clinical material.
- Curriculum and assessment design have become more important and more complex, and medical schools must provide in-house educational expertise.

The relevance of a curriculum

It is worthwhile knowing a little about curriculum development in order to understand the role of clinical teaching. A curriculum is a statement of what is to be learned. It is similar to a road map, in that it indicates a destination, directions for getting there and points along the way for rest, refuelling and reflection on how the journey has gone. The road map analogy is particularly appropriate for clinical attachments, because they are much less structured than a set of lectures and students will generally experience a curriculum in different ways by, for example, doing clinical rotations in different orders. Hence students and clinical teachers need to be mindful of the end point, as well at what may precede or follow the current clinical placement experience.

All training programmes should have some form of documented curriculum, ideally developed with the assistance of a range of stakeholders and interest groups, and therefore reflecting reasonable consensus on what the graduate of the training programme should know and do. Curriculum documents vary considerably in their content, but should contain an overall goal or aim that describes the desired outcome, a set of measurable educational objectives and a description of the entire curriculum. Ideally, the educational processes to be employed throughout the entire course, at least in broad terms, are included.

Clinical teachers do not necessarily need to know the details of a medical school curriculum, but they do need to understand what it is that they will teach. Clinical settings offer particular advantages over classroom settings, in that clinical settings are where all their knowledge, skills and attitudes are applied, with supervision, role modelling and feedback. Hence clinical teaching should focus on helping students learn clinical reasoning, communication, examination, procedural and information management skills within the real world of health-care. A more detailed summary of current curriculum issues, including theoretical aspects, can be found in Chapter 7.

Helping learners with different levels of experience

Clinical teaching can be applied to learners at different levels, with different curricula, different expectations and different needs of learners at each level. This book is primarily about teaching medical students, who need to follow their curriculum and will not need to know as much detail as training registrars. The obvious point is not to treat students and registrars as if they have the same learning needs. Just as paediatrics is not 'mini-adult medicine', teaching medical students is not just 'mini-registrar' teaching.

Medical school curricula now often place students in clinical placements earlier than many clinical teachers are used to, and at several different levels. For example, first-year students may attend for communication skills practice, middle-year students for basic examination skills coaching, and senior students for complete patient work-ups. Clearly, these are quite different tasks and clinical teachers must tailor their approach to the needs of the particular group.

Another variation on this theme is consideration of whether students from graduate entry programmes have different learning needs to those from undergraduate entry programmes (although graduates do sometimes enter these programmes). This is a concern for some clinical teachers who are involved with students from more than one medical school. Graduate course students all have a prior university degree. In theory, they are often a little older, their backgrounds more diverse, their motivation to study medicine more mature and their independent learning skills better than students in undergraduate entry courses.

In practice, anecdotal reports suggest there may be other differences. From the perspective of teaching and learning, graduate entry students may be more likely to use an independent, resource-based learning approach, and be more assertive than school-leavers. On the other hand, some observers feel that graduate entry students may have more shallow biomedical science knowledge and more clinical experience, because they have studied biomedical science either less or some time ago. Some teachers find the assertiveness to be a challenge, interpreting it as disrespect, when it might just reflect a better understanding of personal learning needs and the confidence to express it. Attendance of older students (graduate entry or not) can be affected by their greater need to work and earn money; older students are more likely to have partners and children, and therefore competing responsibilities. Scheduling part-time work is difficult around changing clinical placement requirements during the academic year, so it is worth discussing timing of teaching activities if there is scope for flexibility. Younger school-leavers are more likely to attend as directed, but they pose other challenges to medical school staff early in the course as they travel the journey to mature adulthood.

The final learning objectives of all medical courses are very similar, due to the influence of the licensing bodies (Medical Boards or Councils), and clinical teaching, in particular that during senior years, should be much the same regardless of the curriculum philosophy. There will be greater difference during more junior years (the actual year may be different in the variety of four-, five- and six-year courses). However, there may be as many differences between students from similar schools with either graduate or undergraduate entry criteria as between schools with different entry criteria. A comparison of possible attributes of graduate entry and undergraduate entry students is summarised in Box 2.2.

Box 2.2 Attributes of graduate entry and undergraduate entry medical students

Graduate entry programme
- All have prior degrees.
- More have had prior careers and broader life experiences.
- More older students.
- More mature decision and motivation to study medicine.
- More distant biomedical science?
- More used to resource based learning?
- More assertive about needs?

Undergraduate entry programme
- A minority have prior degrees.
- Fewer have had prior life experience outside school.
- Fewer older students.
- Decision to study medicine made at a younger age.
- More recent biomedical science?
- More used to didactic teaching?
- More accepting of what is offered?

Student learning

Learning is a natural phenomenon, and motivated, academically able medical students will learn almost despite what medical schools and clinical teachers do.

This does not mean, however, that clinical teachers should not consider ways of facilitating, or at least not obstructing, the learning of their students.

Preferred learning styles

Learners learn differently according to personality characteristics and experience. Take a moment to think about your own preferred learning methods. Do you remember more after reading, being told what to do by a more senior colleague, listening to audiotapes, watching videotapes or by just 'doing'? On balance, most health professionals tend to prefer to learn from interaction and discussion with colleagues and from practising new skills in clinical practice, just happy to watch what happens and then learn from doing. Others, particularly those in academic practice and certain specialist groups, tend to prefer reading journals and books, needing to understand why certain things happen – a more analytical approach. Learning styes are almost certainly unrelated to clinical competence and perform-ance, although may be related to ultimate career choice.

While formal measurement of learning styles is not particularly helpful, there is a simple exercise that teachers and learners can do to raise mutual awareness of how they prefer to learn. The *Learning Styles Questionnaire* (*see* Further reading) is a simple 10-minute, self-scoring exercise that, if done honestly, can help indi-viduals to understand their preferred learning style. The questionnaire results should not be taken too seriously, but rather used as a discussion point. Perhaps the real power of such an exercise is where a group of learners and the teacher share their results. Often the most significant mismatch is not amongst the students, but between the teacher and the students. Teachers are likely to present information for students in a way that suits the teachers' personal learning styles, meaning that academics often present information with detailed, pedantic discussions of the theory, embellished with comments based on personal research experience, when many students are switched off by this and just want to hear the pithy, practical summary.

The point is that no learning style is necessarily better than any other and teachers should try to match their delivery to the learning styles of their students. There will be some within-group and between-group variations, so this needs to be considered with every new group of students. Try to look for signs – for example, a student who regularly 'switches off' during detailed theoretical discussions – and then help students to do what works for them.

Responsibility for learning

Teachers undoubtedly have responsibility for teaching, but learning is not guaranteed even where responsible teachers do their jobs well. Learners are responsible for their own learning, particularly as they progress to the more senior years of a medical course. How this balance evolves depends in part on the behaviour of teachers.

Traditional didactic teaching – cruelly called the 'jug to mug' approach – involves teachers telling learners what to learn. This has its place, particularly with more junior learners, but is not popular with educationalists because it does little to encourage learners to work out what they need to learn and there is evidence that such knowledge is not retained for long.

This is where the concept of adult learning becomes prominent. Conceptually, adult learning means allowing learners greater choice of, and control over, what and how they will learn. Adult learners are regarded as experienced in life, knowing what they need to learn, and with prior experiences that can facilitate learning. They should be able to commence an educational programme that is relevant to past experiences, current level of knowledge and future directions. Learning is essentially experiential, based on prior knowledge, understanding and experience. Adult learners are known to: value learning; take responsibility for their learning; receive feedback on their performance; enjoy being challenged to solve problems relevant to future roles; value time for reflection and independent learning; and learn from mistakes.

Most medical schools assume that their students will behave as adult learners. There may be some differences in learning behaviour between graduate entry and school-leaver entry students: in classical adult learning theory graduate entry students are more mature and therefore more proficient at adult learning. However, there is some controversy over what this concept means at different ages, as the original thinking around adult learning was based on adults attending night classes, learning what they wanted in a less formal environment. Medical courses are far more formal, with relatively few optional subjects and a huge amount of information to manage, if not learn. The most important determinant of the learning strategies of students may in fact be the curriculum delivery model. Learning may well be more effective at all stages in life when the learner is motivated and the course is enjoyable. Hence curricula should adopt small group processes, include early clinical experience, and make the curriculum relevant to clinical practice. The most common, but not the only, approach that includes these features is problem-based learning (PBL).

The term 'self-directed learning' is also frequently mentioned in curriculum documents and discussions. A concept related to adult learning, it means that responsible learners will be able over a prolonged career to work out and address their learning needs. While all medical courses will list in their goals the production of self-directed learners, it is unwise to assume that medical students are able to or even should do this, particularly in the earlier years of the course. All medical curricula in fact guide student learning very deliberately towards expected outcomes, although most encourage students to develop the capacity to be self-directed learners by graduation, as less structure and guidance is provided at the postgraduate level.

Negotiating learning needs

One consequence of the adult leaning concept, where learners take increasing responsibility for their learning, is that learners must contribute to decisions about what they should learn. This decision should be based on a combination of what the course designers and teachers believe that learners should learn and what learners have already achieved. With the increasing diversity of student back-grounds, some will know more than others. Hence part of taking responsibility is a commitment to negotiate learning activities that satisfy both course require-ments and individual learner needs.

This concept works better at postgraduate levels, when individuals might be more confident of what they know or do not know and feel less constrained by having to follow a set curriculum, but is becoming increasingly relevant with older and graduate students. For example, a student with an Honours Bachelor degree in Anatomy almost certainly does not need to do the anatomy parts of a medical course (often at a lower level in newer curricula), but may well make an excellent tutor for more junior medical students.

Most medical schools ask students to maintain some form of learning portfolio to document learning progress and assist in identifying gaps, but this works better with experienced professionals in continuing professional development. It can also work with younger medical students, particularly those in the more senior years, but with increased guidance. Learning portfolios are discussed further in Chapter 5.

Impact of the teaching delivery model

A hotly debated issue is how to sequence so-called 'basic' and more advanced knowledge and skills during a curriculum. In other words, what (if any) 'building blocks' must be delivered in a didactic manner to enable learners to be more actively involved in determining personal learning needs. This is the centre of many debates about medical curricula. For example, should students study anatomy and biochemistry, etc. before clinical medicine? If so, this could result in a rather didactic programme full of lectures. Lectures are often criticised but are not necessarily poor educationally. While they are a rather weak form of delivering straight factual content, they can be very effective at delivering a current and concise perspective on a complex topic by a skilled presenter.

An alternative method is PBL and all of the hybrid courses that have since developed. These mostly have in common the integration of basic and clinical science curriculum strands and themes into simulated clinical cases. Well-constructed PBL cases can encourage learners to discover knowledge and skills that are relevant to the clinical scenario. Students can learn from each other, from staff members, or from library and other resources. There is some evidence that knowledge is remembered better this way, as it is recalled when learners are confronted later by similar clinical scenarios, and there is no evidence that students know less at the end of a PBL course than do those of more traditional courses. A further potential advantage of newer curricula is that they might produce more self-directed learners, but there is little evidence to support this. The PBL approach may not be as effective in clinical settings as there students can learn from several encounters with real patients, but the principles of inquiry inherent in PBL are still useful.

Another method places still more responsibility on learners, with learners being given access to a wide range of resources, time to pursue individual or group learning objectives, and formative assessment to provide feedback on their progress.

In reality, most medical school programmes use a combination of methods that include didactic, PBL and more autonomous self-learning characteristics at particular points. The level of responsibility placed on learners should increase through the course and reach a high level in the senior years.

Achieving the desired depth of learning

One of the more subtle, yet extremely important, curriculum issues to understand is the depth of learning that is required of learners. This can best be understood by thinking of a list of clinical issues that medical students are likely to encounter during a clinical rotation – for example, asthma, diabetes and hypertension. All are common and important conditions that medical practitioners are likely to deal with for their entire clinical careers. However, whereas it is relatively easy to define the level of knowledge and understanding needed for competent graduates licensed for independent practice, it is less easy to define for students how much they need to know, and not to know, at their stage of professional development. For example, novice clinical students may need to know the pathology, how to gather relevant information from history and examination, and a list of possible diagnoses. Slightly more senior students may need to know that plus details of relevant diagnostic testing and simple management information.

A related aspect occurs in integrated curricula, where subject material is usually not presented in a linear fashion, but rather entwined with material from other subjects. This can make more difficult the task of knowing just how much of each entwined subject the learner should master.

The desired depth of learning required is best illustrated to learners in two ways. The first is through carefully worded learning objectives, as these should state clearly whether it is information gathering, diagnostic or management skills that are necessary. The second is through formative assessment, where trial questions (with answers) guide learners about how much should be learned. Depth indicators are discussed more in Chapters 5 and 7.

Student–teacher relationships

A method commonly used in clinical teaching is a form of 'apprenticeship' – often called a 'clerkship' in North America – to more experienced clinicians. This often combines a less explicitly defined curriculum, learning by watching the 'master', performing tasks under supervision until competence is reached, and then assuming an increasing degree of responsibility. Teachers are the 'masters', passing on applied experiential wisdom, guiding and nurturing learning. While this model has evolved and has been incorporated with more formal teaching methods in more recent curricula, the relationship between learners and their teachers remains crucial to the success of clinical teaching.

The nature of student–teacher relationships is therefore worthy of consideration. Students and teachers do not have to be friends; indeed, that is unlikely where the student is 20 and the clinical teacher is 40 – a near generational age gap. Students may become friends of registrars and registrars may become friends of consultants, in a more typical collegial manner seen amongst experienced professionals. What is necessary at all stages is mutual respect for the different roles. Students expect good teaching and teachers expect attentive learning, both of which are professional rather than personal transactions. Clinical teachers sometimes have unrealistic expectations of much more junior learners, who will not necessarily want to become over-friendly, but rather get to the next stage and move on.

Where the relationship is strong, learning can be quick and enjoyable, perhaps resulting in long-term, career-influencing friendships (*see* role modelling, p. 35). However, one of the weaknesses of such a close relationship is that sometimes teachers and learners do not get on well. The most common causes are a clash of personalities or a student or teacher having personal or health problems. Personality clashes are not a fault of either the supervisor or the learner, although a record of several similar clashes might lead course organisers to conclude that the most frequently involved person (teacher or learner) has a deeper problem that might need to be explored and addressed. The more difficult problems are usually due to poor attitudes or mental health concerns.

Clinical teachers need to be aware of their own personality and preferred learning style and should develop a capacity to at least make an educated guess at the same attributes of their students. Sometimes just possessing this awareness allows for some simple adjustments that lead to an improvement in the relationship. If not, a frank discussion with the student might achieve mutual awareness and therefore mutual avoidance of misunderstanding. Should this fail, course organisers should be involved, as any relationship between a teacher and a learner involves an obvious imbalance of power within the educational organisation and carries some risk of a student complaint. The main responsibility for taking action rests with the clinical teacher, although learners should also be encouraged to report problems to the course organiser. Sometimes the best course of action is a 'no fault' changing of group allocations to avoid potentially quite destructive relationships that hinder the learner's progress and/or the clinical teacher's enthusiasm.

Organising clinical teaching

One of the key determinants of the success of clinical teaching is its organisation. This has two aspects. The first is how to schedule teaching activities, in both time and location. The second is the orientation of the clinical unit to be a teaching unit, ideally through the development of a teaching plan for the clinical unit.

Teaching and learning activities need to be carefully scheduled to minimise competition between clinical and teaching duties. One of the realities of busy clinical settings is that when clinical duties and teaching duties compete for time, clinical duties usually take priority. This is understandable and appropriate whenever patient care requires an urgent intervention to save a life, but is less acceptable for non-urgent situations. Should teaching come off second best too often, the quality of teaching programmes falls and teachers feel under more pressure than is necessary or healthy. The answer lies in how both activities are scheduled. Teaching sessions for core tutorial topics should not be arranged for times when the clinical teacher is on call for urgent admissions or ward calls, but rather during 'ordinary' clinical time that is 'protected' from urgent distractions. Teaching can still occur during times on call for urgent problems, but this should be more focused on the patients being dealt with and how they exemplify the core teaching, and therefore be more experiential and *ad hoc*.

A related issue is the location of the teaching. Ideally, this should take place close to patient care, on ward rounds and in clinics, etc. Many clinical units now have their own tutorial rooms adjacent to clinical areas, so student tutorials and case presentations can be held within the clinical unit. The more students are made to feel part of the healthcare team, the better.

Clinical organisations in healthcare facilities should, if they take their teaching role seriously, develop a plan that helps staff and students to get the most educational value from clinical placements. Such a plan could include information such as that in Box 2.3. This information is useful for inculcating an academic culture in the organisational unit and to attract like-minded staff and even students (if they have a choice of unit) on the basis of the quality of the clinical and educational experience.

Box 2.3 Useful information for inclusion in an organisational teaching plan

- Descriptions of the organisation: location; layout; staff; contacts; access and service provision arrangements.
- Descriptions of the patient problems seen, relationships to other organisational units, common clinical conditions managed.
- Descriptions of teaching resources available in the organisational unit: staff responsible for teaching; their clinical and educational interests; library and internet access, etc.
- Strengths and opportunities offered by the organisational unit to learners, e.g. renal medicine, women's health, palliative care, etc. This information should reflect practice and staff profiles.
- How teaching and learning is organised in the practice. For example, what teaching methods are used, when and how often clinical teachers and students meet, who is available to assist with particular needs, etc.
- What assessments are conducted within the organisation or term and how they are conducted.

Organisation is also useful for individual teaching sessions. A sound move is to prepare a teaching session plan for every teaching session, at either the individual or unit level, or both. This does not have to be followed obsessionally, as clinical teaching often depends on the clinical material (i.e. patients) available at the time, but the constant issues should be documented to guide presentation and ensure coverage of the curriculum. This is particularly important if the usual clinical teacher is not available and another has to step in and conduct the session without the benefit of the original clinical teacher's memory. A list of information that should be included in a teaching session plan is included in Box 2.4.

Box 2.4 Useful information for inclusion in an individual teaching session plan

- Session title and objective.
- Links to curriculum (domain, subject, year level, etc.).
- Specific learning objectives to be covered.
- Expected learning outcomes of session for the students.

Continued

> - Resources needed (patients, models, slides, co-tutors, etc.).
> - How will teacher know the session has achieved its objectives.

Teaching and learning in action

Following chapters provide details on a range of practice-based teaching methods. These include how to exploit the range of current clinical settings, such as ward rounds, clinics, same-day services, procedural sessions and primary care services. All of these methods employ common principles of clinical teaching, summarised as follows.

- Learning should occur in the context of real clinical encounters. Initially this can (and perhaps should, for safety reasons) be in simulated clinical settings, but should include genuine clinical care settings. Knowledge without application is relatively useless. This is the basis of 'case-based' teaching and learning. Learners will remember better when they are able to think back to past examples. The more they see and learn, the more diagnoses will be based on elaborated knowledge (pattern matching) rather than hypothetico-deductive thinking (*see* Chapter 7). Expertise is built through experience.
- Learning can choose its own time to happen, in two ways. The first is where learners experience 'ah-ha' moments, where the penny drops and a vague swirl of ideas becomes a concept. Experienced teachers will recognise when this occurs and should seize the opportunity to reinforce the learning. Asking the student to verbalise their revelation might help others as well as themselves. The second is where the teacher recognises an opportunity to help learners focus on, or understand, something important that just arises unexpectedly. For example, when discussing a young adult patient with rather brittle diabetes, why not include a brief discussion of the ethics of renewing the patient's driving licence? This concept is known as 'the teachable moment' and should also be seized if time allows.
- Learning should be inquiry-based. Experience alone is not enough. Experience will generate questions for which learners seek answers. However, learners will remember better when they personally discover information and skills relevant to their practice. Supervisors should resist the temptation to provide quick answers to questions. It is often better to turn the question back to the learner, suggesting that they find out the answer and tell you at a future appointment. This is the 'educational prescription' concept developed by David Sackett about 20 years ago. His practice, in response to a student's question about a clinical case, was to write on a piece of paper (a bit like a prescription for medication) the question to be answered and the time the answer was to be delivered. Sometimes he wrote the prescription to himself, demonstrating that even experienced clinicians had to look up information to answer such questions (great role modelling!). While perhaps not needing to be quite so formal, the concept is useful.
- Learning should be reflective. The term 'reflection' can be scary for some, but it really means that learners need to cycle mentally through the process of getting information that helps answer their questions and then deciding how

well their questions have been answered. Should the information not seem sufficient, then further information should be sought through literature searches, further clinical experience, or asking more experienced colleagues. Where possible, answers should be evidence-based, just as with clinical medical practice. Learners should also be encouraged to question themselves often, and seek answers to those questions.

- Learning is driven by feedback on one's own performance. Clinical teachers need to be skilled in giving feedback to their learners. In summary, the rules are: be specific, timely and positive, and couch feedback in terms of comments or questions, as that promotes reflection. Being positive can be difficult when the feedback is critical, but even critical feedback should be accompanied by some positive comment, ideally before and after the criticism. Asking questions of learners is a powerful way of providing feedback and directing learning.
- Learning should be supported by a range of relevant and useful educational resources that are held within the practice. Some suggestions for a teaching practice 'library' are provided in Appendix 2, and include books, journals and web access.
- Learning needs to be reinforced, again and again. This is one role of assessment processes, and this explains one of the advantages of frequent formative assessment.
- Learning should involve longitudinal involvement in clinical care across different sectors of healthcare. One of the emerging trends in modern healthcare is greater integration of community and hospital-based care. With attachments that cross primary and secondary care 'barriers', the concept of continuity of care can be understood from personal experience. A simple technique is to attach learners to patients who are referred both from primary care into specialist or hospital care, and vice versa. Participating in the whole healthcare experience of patients – from presentation, through investigations, referral, treatment and back home – can be a valuable learning experience.
- Learning occurs through role modelling. This is remarkably powerful. Just as Michael Balint spoke of the doctor as the 'drug', meaning that doctors can have profound effects on their patients, supervisors can have profound effects on their learners. Clinicians often talk about particular individuals who had a profound influence on their careers. Ideally, supervisors should demonstrate a reflective, inquiry-based learning style to their learners; this role-models good learning behaviour for the next generation of teachers.

Technical skills

Just as the practice of medicine is becoming more technology-assisted, so too is education. The implication for clinical teachers is that they need to know how to use simple computer software and hardware if they are going to teach students.

It used to be easy – just to turn up at the appointed time with a carousel of slides from one's personal collection, place the carousel on the slide projector and press start. Well, it wasn't always quite that easy, as carousels sometimes jammed or the slides were accidentally inserted back-to-front or upside down!

Now, however, clinical teachers can be helped (or hindered) by seminar room consoles that link computers, DVDs, VCRs, video-conferencing equipment, CD players and television sets. To paraphrase the old adage, when the technology works it is very, very good, and when it does not, it is horrid!

Some institutions have resident technicians to do this, but many do not. Therefore the modern clinical teacher needs to be familiar with current technology and should always arrive 10–15 minutes early for sessions that require its use, so that the equipment can be test-run. Technical glitches will occur, especially in seminar rooms being used by many different groups, and it usually takes only a few minutes to diagnose and fix simple problems. Better to do this before than after commencement time! The medical school or teaching hospital should be able to provide the necessary simple training.

The other aspect is the use of modern software to create a presentation. It is possible to blend still images, moving images, sound and text in innovative ways, but if this is overdone, the audience may not notice the central messages of the presentation. This issue is discussed more in Chapter 3.

Summary

This chapter has provided an overview of the development and current context of clinical teaching and learning, primarily for medical students. Some key concepts are summarised as a precursor to the next three chapters, in Part 2, which are written from a very practical perspective, using scenarios to provoke consideration of applying educational theory in day-to-day clinical teaching practice. A deeper exploration of the educational theory underpinning this material is provided in Part 3.

Further reading

- Bligh JD (1993) The S-SLDRS: a short questionnaire about self-directed learning. *Postgraduate Education for General Practice.* **4**: 255–6.
  This describes an interesting exercise for self-assessment of learning styles and methods. Potentially useful to help clinical teachers understand their students and themselves.
- CanMEDS 2000 (2000) Extract from the CanMEDS 2000 Project Societal Needs Working Group Report. *Medical Teacher.* **22**: 549–54.
  A clear explanation of the broader roles of medical practitioners. Similar documents now exist for almost all medical boards.
- Lewis AP and Bolden KJ (1989) General practitioners and their learning styles. *Journal of the Royal College of General Practitioners.* **39**(322): 187–9.
  This describes the use of learning styles questionnaires with general practitioners and other health professionals, most of whom desire relevance and efficiency in their learning. Hospital-based clinical teachers are probably similar in their pragmatism. On the other hand, academic clinicians who design curricula may be more analytical and therefore tend to develop educational programmes that appeal to learning styles similar to their own. Completing this questionnaire may help clinical teachers understand where they lie in the spectrum of learning styles.
- McLeod PJ, Steinert Y, Meagher T *et al.* (2003) The ABCs of pedagogy for clinical teachers. *Medical Education.* **37**: 638–44.
  Research-derived list of core pedagogic concepts that might improve clinical teaching.
- Sackett DL *et al.* (2000) *Evidence-Based Medicine. How to practice and teach EBM.* Churchill Livingstone, Edinburgh.

Part 2

Clinical teaching practice

Chapter 3

Clinical teaching skills

> It is for life, not for school, that we learn.
>
> Seneca, 4 BC–65AD

Introduction

Just as being a sound clinician requires a set of clinical skills – the ability to take a history, conduct a physical examination, clinical reasoning and planning evidence-based management – being a sound clinical teacher requires a set of educational skills that enhance knowledge acquisition by, and skills transfer to, learners. Educationalists call these teaching *microskills*. Where possible, these should be evidence-based (that is, based on the findings of educational research). Few are innate and all can be learned by clinicians who want to become better teachers.

This chapter presents a series of clinical teaching microskills, where possible including scenarios, all based on genuine events, that exemplify their use. A suggested way of using these scenarios is, after reading each of them, to jot down some thoughts about the learning process that was going on. Answering the following questions may be a useful guide.

1   What techniques did the clinical teacher use?
2   How well would the learners have been motivated, engaged and able to learn?
3   Who got the most out of the encounter?
4   How could learning have been improved?

The guest lecture

Clinicians are often invited to contribute their expertise in the form of a lecture. This is a familiar format and all clinicians are experienced receivers of lectures. Many enjoy being asked to do this, as it is recognition that they are knowledgeable and important to the medical school programme. Lectures can be a highly efficient way of delivering synthesised information. When done well, they are engaging and can provide information that has meaning to the listeners. However, it is so easily done poorly.

Scenario 3.1

Dr A had a national reputation for being an expert in his field and travelled the nation delivering guest lectures. Organisers would announce forthcoming events with pride, telling students, registrars and experienced doctors that they should feel honoured to be included in the itinerary as

---

his interactive style made the lectures fun. After brief introductions, the presentation began. It consisted of a series of slides of 'spot diagnoses', but sometimes not classic presentations, with limited clinical information. Instead of telling the audience the answers, the speaker would ask the audience to provide them. Sometimes this happened quickly, with usually the more experienced members of the audience being right. If somebody suggested the wrong answer they were made fun of, and soon fewer people were brave enough to make a suggestion. If nobody could recognise the condition, or perhaps did not have the confidence to shout it out, the speaker would become frustrated, pointing to people in the front row for answers and, when they were incorrect, announced that the profession in this part of the world was not very bright. After flashing 50–60 slides, with less and less discussion on each slide, the lecturer was thanked. The few experts left the room with heads held high, because their expertise had been affirmed, but most left with a sense of relief and a sense that they could never know much about that subject.

Scenario 3.2

Dr B was a busy clinician who knew a lot about the topic and had agreed to put together a presentation to facilitate student education. He did a 'cut and paste' from presentations he had given to registrars and to colleagues at a conference, and ended up with 90 slides of detailed information. Several of these were images of clinical conditions, as he knew that students liked clinical material and also that the more people see images the more likely they are to recognise them later. He was aware that he was presenting more information than the students really needed (according to their curriculum), but he felt that the curriculum was too shallow in his discipline area and that a bit extra would not hurt. He turned down the lights so that the students could see the images better. He felt as if he had to really rush through the slides to finish on time, but after 55 minutes the next class was hammering on the door to be let in, and he had still not finished. This was very frustrating as he felt he had not got across all his intended messages.

Scenario 3.3

Dr C had prepared the presentation very carefully, following the curriculum closely. She felt proudly that this was perhaps her best ever lecture, as she had included a lot of additional information that elaborated on the core information. The presentation consisted of about 40 slides, each with about six or seven dot-points. To fit these in, she had used font size 18 and they were a bit hard to read from the back of the room, but she readily apologised for this and provided a handout containing the complete presentation, as well as placing the presentation on the school's website. She then read every slide very carefully, finishing precisely on time.

Scenario 3.4

Dr D knew that she really could not discuss all the issues relevant to the topic in only 50 minutes. She chose instead to prepare a relatively shallow overview of the key issues in a series of about 25 slides, each of which had three or four dot-points. She then verbally elaborated around the issues, asking for questions at key points to ensure the students were on task. Before closing, she provided a list of important issues for students to pursue, some suggested readings, and her email address for them to ask any questions.

Scenario 3.5

Dr E knew that she really could not discuss all the issues relevant to the topic in only 50 minutes, and she knew from experience that students become anxious if they feel that examinable material is not fully explained. She therefore chose to prepare two versions of her presentation. One was loaded onto the school's website – a summary of the key issues in a series of about 20 slides, each of which had three or four dot-points, all in black and white (to minimise download times). Students were encouraged to access this, to add to it what they learned from the lecture, the readings and discussion amongst themselves, and then print their own version of detailed notes based on the summary. She also prepared a more detailed colour version that was slightly longer and more attractive, and during the lecture verbally elaborated around the issues, asking for questions at key points to ensure the students were grasping the issues. The second to last slide consisted of the key learning points for the lecture, and the final slide listed recommended readings and discussion points. She also suggested a one-hour period in three days' time when she would be in her office to help students who were having trouble mastering the issues.

Scenario 3.1 illustrates the challenge of presenting a lecture to an audience of individuals with a range of expertise from very high to very low. Keeping all of them engaged and learning is extremely difficult. The experts may feel validated and occasionally challenged, but the novices are likely to feel overwhelmed by the fast pace. In Chapter 7 you will find a section on clinical reasoning, or how we process complex information to achieve a diagnosis. This shows that students will try to use hypothetico-deductive reasoning in the absence of sufficient information, whereas the teachers are likely to be pattern matching. Another feature is the singling out of people to answer questions, the mocking of those who did not know and the comments that other audiences know more. Learners should feel that it is acceptable to try and fail and will clam up and avoid eye contact if they feel under this kind of pressure. In this scenario the real game being played was perhaps self-aggrandisement of the lecturer.

Scenario 3.2 represents a common approach among those who are very busy clinicians and rather inexperienced in education. It highlights the pitfalls of trying to adapt materials from lectures to others, including other levels of learner, and of not practising the lecture to get the timing right. Common errors made by guest lecturers include: not really understanding how the lecture fits into the course; cramming in too much information, much of it at the wrong level for the audience; reading slides instead of talking about them; running out of time and leaving no time for discussion.

Scenario 3.3 illustrates good preparation, but questionable delivery. Presentation slides need a large font size (at least 24) and only three or four bullet points or they will be hard to read and the information too dense for understanding. Further, if everything that needs to be learned is in both the slides and the handouts, why should students attend the lecture? Many lecturers feel that they may not have done their job properly if they have not listed every single relevant fact in their presentation, but it is better to use the lecture to elaborate on, exemplify and explain the factual content. Handouts and lecture notes then become an *aide-mémoire* to that explanation as well as a resource for deeper learning, primed by the presentation.

Scenario 3.4 is both well planned and well delivered. The lecturer focuses on the learning process of the students and works hard at delivering the right amount at digestible intervals. Scenario 3.5 includes some further educationally sound features, such as presenting a different version at the lecture to the notes or web system, and clearly summarising the key learning issues. The former is more interesting and assists in deeper learning, while the latter reassures students who fear missing the point and being disadvantaged in assessment. The offer to be available for further discussion is reasonable, but must have boundaries (time and location), or else teachers can be overwhelmed!

Distilling the messages from these scenarios produces a list of tips for providing better guest lectures; these are summarised in Box 3.1.

Box 3.1 Tips for guest lecturers

- Plan the session very carefully.
- Study the curriculum to make sure you know where your lecture fits in and to ensure that you address the stated learning objectives.
- Be mindful of the level of learner you are addressing and adjust your pitch to their level.
- Use no more than 25–30 slides during a 50-minute session.
- Use font size 24 as a minimum on slides.
- Have no more than four bullet points on a presentation slide.
- Use a limited number of clinical images to place the material in a clinical context and raise interest.
- Use diagrams and figures to summarise complex conceptual issues.
- Never just read the slides: your oral presentation should elaborate the information on them.

- Be animated, move around, ask questions and maintain eye contact with the audience.
- Avoid using too many fancy features (too many colours, sounds, video, etc.) as this may detract from the underlying message.
- Never use a slide that is overcrowded and say 'you probably can't read this as it is too busy . . .' Design slides that are meaningful.
- Carefully observe audience behaviour; adjust your presentation if they look bored or sleepy.
- Avoid turning lights down too far so that you can maintain eye contact with the audience.
- Ensure that you finish in no later than 40 minutes to leave time for questions and discussion.
- Never run over time.
- Provide students with an email address and encourage them to seek clarification when uncertain.

Role modelling

Whether role modeling is something that can be learned is debatable, but this book assumes that all clinical teachers can improve and so will assume that at least awareness of the concept might improve the ability of clinicians to be good role models.

The power of role models, both positive and negative, is probably very large. All of us can remember one or more individuals who inspired us to follow a particular career path, and some of us will also remember at least one individual who turned us off doing something. However, measuring this power is difficult. Consider the following scenarios and work out what is happening.

Scenario 3.6

Dr F was a clinician with a sound reputation for competent medical practice. She seemed to 'know her stuff', and to be well respected by peers and registrars. She enjoyed teaching students and took a group every rotation that she was at work. She always arrived for tutorials and other teaching sessions on time, always stayed until the sessions were over and always covered the curriculum. She related well with students and was known to be a good communicator.

Scenario 3.7

Dr G was a clinician with a reputation for being one of the most brilliant in the local medical community. All the medical people said: 'If you ever get ill,

---

Continued

he's the one to go to!' However, he could be abrasive and judgemental, and he tolerated poorly students who could not answer all of his questions, and so students avoided him if they could. He was also so busy clinically that he was often late for teaching sessions and he spent much of the session time on his mobile phone dealing with urgent clinical business.

Scenario 3.8

Dr H was a gregarious person known to be a sound clinician and eager teacher. However, he often cracked sexually explicit jokes with the students, boasted about his pornographic computer screensavers, and there were rumours that at social events he drank heavily and came on to female students, even if his wife was present.

The message for clinical teachers is to demonstrate as often and consistently as possible the positive attributes of being a sound teaching clinician. The list of attributes is long (*see* Chapter 1), and includes being: a competent clinician, knowledgeable and skilled but aware of personal limits of ability and how to get others with appropriate expertise involved as required in patient care; aware of the needs of the learners in their care; punctual, polite and respectful of patients, other health workers and students; and able to balance professional and personal or family responsibilities. This sounds like an almost superhuman position description, given the dynamics of demanding and competing pressures and the resulting frustrations, but should be the aim of all clinical teachers.

The moral of the story is: if you are to be remembered as a clinical teacher by your students, make sure you are remembered for being a good person, clinician and teacher.

The three scenarios are not far-fetched, as they are based on real people. The obvious question is: who is the best clinical teacher? The obvious answer is Dr F, but unfortunately not all clinical teachers are as saintly as that. Indeed, Dr F may well live an unbalanced life that ignores personal and family needs in order to be such a good teacher. Students are likely to encounter many different kinds of clinical teachers, most more like Dr F than the others, but they will learn from a range of people with different personalities and styles. Clinicians who are too busy to teach, a bit like Dr G, are very commonly encountered, and are probably less dangerous than those who are prone to unprofessional behaviour, like Dr H, who should be removed from the list of clinical teachers. Some tips for being an effective role model are summarised in Box 3.2.

One further aspect of role modelling is dealing with situations where you do not know enough, or make a mistake. Do not try to hide this, but rather openly acknowledge that you need to look up information and perhaps even ask the students to help you. Where a mistake has been made (a lost report, a delay in referral, a prolonged wait, a poorer than expected outcome), apologise and explain the circumstances to patients in the presence of your students. Junior members of the medical profession need to learn how to perform this task as much as the more commonly taught clinical skills.

Box 3.2 Tips for effective role modelling

- Do your best to be a sound clinician, teacher and human being, but aim for the right balance of those demands.
- Be honest, reliable and respectful with patients, colleagues and students.
- Be aware of your limits, be open about them and find ways to make up for them.
- If you cannot make it to a session at short notice, try to contact the students to apologise and to arrange another time.
- Take time for self-care.
- When confronted with a clinical situation that you do not know enough about, make sure that learners see that you acknowledge this and deal with it by seeking the information.
- Demonstrate to learners that you can apologise to patients for delays and errors.

Calibration of expectations

One of the most difficult tasks for novice clinical teachers is to work out the expected level of knowledge, skills and attitudes that medical students in their care should have. The easiest place to start is with the most recent personal experience, usually advanced registrar level. However, judging medical students by the experiences with more mature, more knowledgeable and more experienced people will lead to frustration on the part of both teacher and learner.

Scenario 3.9

Dr I was an eminent clinician with a proud record of both clinical service and training registrars who did well in postgraduate examinations. He preferred not to teach medical students as 'they know so little' and so few were inspired to choose a career in his own discipline area. Students also did not particularly enjoy his teaching, as he asked very hard questions that they felt that even the JHOs and registrars had trouble answering. The theory developed that even if a student answered a question correctly, Dr I would keep asking questions until they could not answer correctly. Dr I was one of the greatest critics of the new medical curriculum because he felt that students knew less than those he had taught in the past.

Most medical students are on a journey towards a long and hopefully rewarding career, but they are close to the beginning of that career pathway. They are younger, interested in exploring the freedoms of young adulthood and university life, will probably not have made a firm decision about career choice, and will obviously know a lot less and be less skilled. The role of the clinical teacher is to help students master the curriculum through exposure to patient care and helping them develop as future professional people.

Some tips for handling this are summarised in Box 3.3. It is wise to put some effort into understanding the requirements of the curriculum of the courses you are involved with (more in Chapter 4). Never assume that medical students from different medical schools or different years of the same medical school have similar learning needs. In particular, never expect a student to know as much as a JHO or a registrar. Some might, but they are rarities. Learning curriculum details can be difficult as curriculum documents are often very long and may be complex, requiring more time than most clinicians have available to understand. The easiest way is to focus on the learning objectives for the particular clinical rotation and the specific year of the course. Some students will exceed these easily or early and you may by negotiation want to try extending their learning, but do not expect students to want to do this.

Box 3.3 Tips for calibrating teaching to learners' needs

- Read and understand at least the curriculum overview and learning objectives of the course in which you are teaching.
- Try to develop an understanding of how learning progresses during the whole course.
- Assuming that students know less than they do is more forgivable than the reverse.
- Start by asking students what they have learned already and how confident they are to tackle the current placement. They will often be modest or under confident, but it defines a place to begin.
- Remember that if students can do a particular rotation either first or last in an academic year (the usual model), they will know more later in the year than earlier. Hence teachers should expect to have to provide different support for first and second-term students, just as they have to with novice registrars.
- Seek opportunities to teach at several levels – junior and senior medical students, interns and registrars, and compare their level of knowledge and understanding.
- Do not worry about recruiting students to your own specialty. Instead, allow them to have a series of positive experiences and later choose what interests them the most.

It is better to be remembered as a clinician who understood learning needs and helped students develop, than as a brilliant clinician whom students tried to avoid.

Observation of learning

Just as learning is a very active cognitive process, so too is observing learners learn. Learning is a complex process, but it is recognisable and measurable.

Experienced teachers can do this almost intuitively, but inexperienced teachers have to work harder to achieve the same understanding. It requires a set of conditions as well as some skill, but the conditions are easy to meet and the skill can be acquired.

What conditions are necessary for learning? Some of this is practical organisation – setting aside undisturbed time in an appropriate location. For example, scheduling case discussions to periods when the clinical teacher is not on call, turning off the mobile phones (everybody's!) and sitting comfortably in a quiet tutorial room to minimise disruption from background noise in a busy ward. Clinical teachers should attempt to empty their minds of thoughts about issues other than the teaching role. I recognise that this is not easy in busy clinical units, but such strategies facilitate learning. Other helpful skills relate to some of the microskills presented in this chapter, including giving appropriate feedback, etc.

How can active learning be recognised? This requires active listening and active observation. Sometimes simple things help, such as good attendance by the learners. In fact, participation in teaching sessions is more important than just being in the room. Teachers often have fun interacting with those students most engaged, when the real focus should be on those who are less engaged. Apparent lack of engagement might be simply due to a different learning style, but it can also mean true disengagement that may be due to an educational or personal problem (*see* later in this chapter).

More subtle and important things to observe include eye contact and movements. Engaged brains will follow conversations with their eyes, flicking them to others, and sometimes up and to the right or left (neuro-linguistic programming suggests this is about accessing memory and constructing ideas). Learners also usually ask questions, particularly the sort of questions that probe and elaborate the discussion. A final set of skills relates to formatively assessing learning progress, a topic that is discussed in more detail in Chapters 5 and 7. Tips for being a more effective observer of learning are summarised in Box 3.4.

Box 3.4 Tips for observing learning

- Take note of attendance, and particularly the participation, of students in teaching activities.
- Minimise potential disruption to teaching sessions (turn off mobile phones, quiet room, avoid on-call periods).
- Maintain focus on the teaching task.
- Carefully monitor attendance and eye contact of learners.
- Monitor the group process.
- Listen carefully to questions that learners ask and to the response to your answers.
- Regularly assess the progress of student learning.

Questioning

The way in which teachers and learners ask and answer questions can have a profound effect on student learning. There is an art, as well as science, to both asking and answering questions.

Asking questions of learners

Questioning is one of the most powerful teaching tools and is accessible by all clinical teachers. One of the commonest errors made by inexperienced teachers is to provide to learners all the information necessary to achieve the learning objectives in a dialogue or set of notes, without discussion. It is the discussion that allows learners to think around the new knowledge, place it in some kind of context, and then store it in deeper knowledge structures.

Scenario 3.10

Dr J began the tutorial with a brief welcome and an announcement that today's topic was renal failure. He then proceeded to give a very detailed and cogent summary of the causes of renal failure, their diagnosis and the broad principles of management. At the end he looked at his watch, asked 'Any questions?' in a way that indicated he did not expect any, and said 'Well if you know all that, you will do well in the exam' and left the students to get on with seeing patients.

Scenario 3.11

Dr K began with a brief welcome and then said: 'Today's topic is renal failure. Have you seen any patients with renal failure yet?' Three students nodded. 'OK, Kayla, could you tell us about the renal failure patient you have seen?' There followed 10 minutes of discussion about the three patients and the group's thoughts on possible causes. After that Dr K said: 'OK. So you already seem to know a bit about this topic. I will just give you a brief rundown on some of the key points – I promise this will be only five minutes, and then we can go back and discuss those three patients and see how much they fit the diagnostic categories.'

Scenario 3.12

A student presented a case of a patient with chest pain during a cardiology tutorial. The history was a rather classical presentation of angina and the student sped through it to get to the physical findings and investigations. The tutor, Dr L, called for a pause and asked the other students in the group: 'So far the history is very typical of angina, but what if the central lower chest pain radiated to the tip of the shoulder blade instead of to the throat?' As the students provided plausible answers, the tutor changed the potential scenario several times, and within a few minutes the differential diagnosis of central acute chest pain had been covered.

The best way to provoke deeper learning is to use the right kind of questions. A very good start is, instead of providing information assumed to be new, to ask learners what they already know about the topic. Do not accept a timid 'not much', but instead provide a clinical scenario in which the new knowledge might be applied and work through the scenario until you feel that you have gone beyond their current knowledge. This helps motivate learners to extend their knowledge and also provides a degree of tailoring of teaching to individual needs. Next, start providing the new knowledge, but pause every so often and check their understanding. Here, instead of asking 'Have you all got that?' (the almost universal responses are a nod or a mumbled 'yes'), ask the learners to summarise what has been covered so far. This reiteration helps firm up the memory and understanding. Involve all learners in the summarising and ask questions that explore meaning and understanding, such as 'And how would you apply that in a case of a patient with . . .?'

This approach is more interesting and more effective for most learners. The only real disadvantage is that it is more time-consuming than the straight, didactic lecture model. Also, some experienced clinicians may be uncomfortable with the questioning approach as they feel it threatens their authority and does not recognise their extensive knowledge, but can be reassured that this is not the way that learners view expertise. It is possible to be both a great and wise clinician and a wise teacher.

Another valuable style of questioning is 'what if' questions that raise hypothetical situations that make students think in different directions. Scenario 3.12 illustrates an example, where the tutor turned a rather obvious clinical history into a discussion of differential diagnoses if symptoms were a little different. The same technique can be applied to change examination findings ('What if the liver was enlarged?') and investigation results ('What if the ESR had come back at 100?'). This technique is also very useful for case presentations where the clinical history is either not very revealing or is relatively normal. Careful changes to the symptoms by using 'what if' questions can lead students into a much broader and useful discussion about clinical pathology, even where the patient turns out not to have any such pathology.

Some suggestions for using questions are summarised in Box 3.5.

Box 3.5 Questions as teaching tools

- Ask what learners already know before adding new knowledge.
- Seek to clarify each learner's current depth of knowledge and understanding.
- Periodically check understanding by asking learners to summarise what they have heard.

Continued

- Regularly link new material to clinical cases that learners have seen or may see.
- Extend discussion of cases by asking 'what if' questions.

Answering learners' questions

A related issue is the question of how best to respond to questions from learners. Good clinical teachers encourage learners to ask questions that clarify or elaborate knowledge and understanding. The way they respond to these questions can help learners think again and learn more. In particular, it is possible to help learners see how to apply new knowledge in clinical situations, with patients they have encountered.

Scenario 3.13

During a case presentation the student paused and asked a question of the clinical teacher: 'Dr M, I looked up how to investigate renal failure and the textbook lists so many options that I could not work out what should be done in this case. Why did this patient have a renal biopsy?' Dr M smiled and gave a quick 10-minute burst on the salient issues in how to investigate renal failure.

Scenario 3.14

During a case presentation the student paused and asked a question of the clinical teacher: 'Dr N, I looked up how to investigate renal failure and the textbook lists so many options that I could not work out what should be done in this case. Why did this patient have a renal biopsy?' Dr N replied, 'Well, what did the textbook say?' When the student replied with a list he had written down, the clinical teacher turned to the other students and asked: 'What do you think? What tests would you order and in what sequence would you order them? What can each test result contribute to your diagnostic reasoning?'

These scenarios demonstrate simply just how different a teaching activity can be when the clinical teacher stops giving simple, direct answers to questions and uses further questions to help learners explore and improve their knowledge and understanding. It is harder work for the learners, but is more effective teaching. Some tips are summarised in Box 3.6.

Box 3.6 Answers as teaching tools

- Avoid answering too many questions directly with factual detail.
- Try to reflect questions back onto the questioner or other learners.
- Link learners' questions back to patients they have seen or might see.

Giving and receiving feedback on performance

Giving feedback is one of the most important roles of a clinical teacher. Learners need to be shown how to perform clinical tasks such as taking histories, conducting physical examinations, etc., have a go at them under observation, receive feedback about their performance and then practise some more; the clinical coaching process. The quality of the feedback can have a powerful affect on learning.

Scenario 3.15

At the end of the third week of an eight-week clinical placement, one student was asked to stay behind when the group was dismissed after the tutorial. With little preamble, Dr O said: 'I need to let you know that I think you are going to fail the exam at the end of the year. You seem to have important gaps in your knowledge base, compared with the rest of the group, and you do not seem to be getting the message, so I am making it very clear now as a warning. If you do not improve dramatically, you may as well give up now.' The student was stunned, as she had always done quite well in the examinations and she felt that she knew about the same as the others. She plucked up enough courage to ask for more information on the problem, and was told to 'read and memorise [a textbook name] or you will have no hope'. The student left quietly, went home and cried all night, not really understanding either the problem or how to address it.

Scenario 3.16

At the end of the third week of an eight-week clinical placement, Dr P was worried about the learning progress of one student in her group. She emailed this student telling him this and suggesting a time they could meet to discuss her concerns. The student was worried but agreed on a time. At the meeting Dr P began by asking the student how he thought he was progressing. The student had had time to think about things and admitted anxiety at feeling that he was not on top of the curriculum and that his peers appeared to be more knowledgeable. He asked for specific feedback from Dr P on what she thought he was missing and what he could do about it. They then agreed on a plan to do some extra clinical work to broaden his clinical experience and trigger learning in the noted areas of weakness.

Scenario 3.17

The 'teaching round' had been in progress for about 20 minutes, following the usual format. A team of people was moving from bed to bed, seeing all of the patients admitted under the name of the consultant, Dr Q, who with the registrar and the charge nurse made up the front row of the pack. The resident medical officer and intern stood behind, and a group of six medical students were in the back row, barely able to see the patient in the bed they surrounded. The registrar responded first to questions from the consultant, often referring to the JHO and intern for details recorded in the patient's records. The charge nurse knew most about the patient really, but would step in only to correct factual information about the patient's condition. At the back, the students were starting to feel bored and left out, as they were infrequently included in the discussion, apart from an occasional question fired at them by Dr Q, like 'You there on the left! What are the seven causes of hypercalcemia?' Suddenly, Dr Q stopped in mid-sentence, looked at one of the students, and said: 'You there – what is your name? Come closer so I can read your name tag – ah yes, Jones. You know what Jones? You worry me. There is something about you I just can't quite work out. You just stand there quietly, not saying or doing anything. I want you to know that I know what you are up to and will watch you like a hawk for the rest of the term.' With that he resumed his sentence about the patient.

The art of giving educationally sound feedback lies in following some simple principles or rules. First, feedback is more easily received when the learner is comfortable with the teacher. Hence things go better when there is a reasonably positive relationship between the two participants. It often helps to allow the student to observe and comment on the performance of the teacher; this reminds both participants that learning is a two-way process. Second, feedback should begin with positive comments (there should always be some to make!), proceed through issues that might be a concern, and finish with positive comments. Overly negative feedback without any positive comment can come over as very harsh, even intimidating. Third, feedback should be constructive, with comments about what could be improved, rather than direct criticism. Fourth, feedback should be specific, in that issues are identified precisely. For example, commenting that the student's body language was 'inappropriate' is less helpful than commenting on eye contact, position across a desk, or sitting back instead of forward, etc., if one of those was the specific concern. Fifth, feedback should be timely, in the sense of being as soon as possible after the observation, rather than several days later. Finally, often the best way to raise an issue is to ask the learner to comment on their own performance, as learners will often be strongly self-critical and are likely to raise issues identified by the teacher anyway. Ideally, the learner should be invited to make comments on their performance before the teacher does.

Back to the scenarios, where we should assume that in both the tutor had reasonable grounds for the concerns. In the first 'giving feedback' scenario (3.15), the tutor provides non-specific, non-constructive and untimely feedback without really engaging the learner. Indeed, it may have embarrassed the learner in front of her peers, did not necessarily achieve her acceptance that there is a problem, left her stranded without a real plan to improve, and risked demotivating the learner. It is an example of teaching by *intimidation* by a tutor who does not understand educational practice. In the second, the tutor provides confidential, specific and constructive feedback with an offer to help. In neither scenario is the feedback necessarily timely, as in soon after specific observed behaviours. However, they were both timely in the sense that such feedback should be given after sufficient time to observe and make a judgement, but with sufficient time left to do something about it.

Some tips for providing educationally sound feedback are listed in Box 3.7. For further information on giving feedback, read *The Consultation* by Pendleton *et al.* which, although 20 years old and written for postgraduate GP education, is highly relevant to all forms of clinical teaching.

Box 3.7 Tips for providing educationally sound feedback

- Be positive at both the start and finish.
- Invite the learner to go first.
- Make comments rather than judgements.
- Be as specific as possible.
- Be as timely as possible.
- Discuss how things might be done next time.
- Agree on a plan for improvement and review.

Clinical skills coaching

This is one of the most important roles of clinical teachers, as clinical skills can really be learned best with real patients and in real clinical settings. There are, however, three steps to the process. The first is to demonstrate clearly the right way to perform a particular clinical skill. For example, if students are being taught how to physically examine a chest, commence with a verbal description of what to do and then either show a video of an experienced clinician doing it correctly or conduct an examination on a real patient, a simulated patient or even one of the students. Using students is acceptable for non-intimate and non-invasive procedures, so long as the student consents, but it is probably better to use either a simulated or consenting real patient.

One of the key skills required is the ability to 'let the learner be free' to learn from their mistakes in a safe environment. This requires a self-confident clinical teacher who knows what novice learners can do, and who can trust learners to do their best and not overextend themselves. In such a controlled situation safety should be assured.

Box 3.8 Steps in clinical skill development

1 Describe the skill to be developed.
2 Demonstrate the 'correct' method to learners.

Continued

3 Observe the learners perform the skill on a model or a simulated patient and give constructive feedback, and repeat it until they can perform it safely.
4 Allow learners to perform the skill with a real patient and give constructive feedback.
5 If performance is OK, allow learners to continue to perform the skill on real patients with decreasing levels of supervision as mastery is achieved.
6 For some skills performed infrequently learners may need to return to step 3.

Once students have seen it done and have thought through how to perform the skill, the second step is to ask the student to perform the skill on a patient model or simulated patient (or a real one, or possibly a fellow student). The range and quality of patient models is improving every week, so it may soon become possible to simulate most or all of the common procedures. Carefully observe and offer feedback. Once the student appears to have achieved safety (particularly important for procedural skills or examination skills that may be sensitive or possibly painful), the third step is to allow the student to perform the procedure or skills under observation on a real patient and provide feedback, as well as asking the patient to provide feedback. Once the student is thought to have performed the procedure or skills to a satisfactory standard, he or she then practises it many times on real patients under decreasingly active observation. This process is summarised in Box 3.8. Please note that this is *not* the 'see one, do one, teach one' approach that is the butt of jokes!

Setting 'homework': use of flexible time

Most curricula in modern medical schools schedule formal teaching activities for only about half of the week, or around 20 hours at a maximum. These activities include teaching rounds, clinics, procedural sessions and tutorials.

What about the other half of the week? This should be regarded not as 'free' time, but 'flexible' time, during which students should still be engaged in learning, but in individual or informal group settings. This includes time for library research, following patients through the healthcare system, working up case presentations, practising examination and procedural skills, etc. Many students need guidance in order to utilise this time effectively and some structure imposed by clinical teachers can be a positive thing.

Scenario 3.18

During the case presentation the student asked the clinical teacher, Dr R: 'Dr R, why did this patient have a renal CT first instead of a renal ultrasound?' Dr R explained this quickly and the discussion moved on to another topic.

Scenario 3.19

During the case presentation the student asked the clinical teacher, Dr S: 'Dr S, why did this patient have a renal CT first instead of a renal ultrasound?' Dr S reflected this back as a question to the whole group of students. When none could provide an explanation, Dr S asked the student who asked the question of him to find the answer later and report back at Friday's tutorial with the answer. The student went to the library and found a review article on renal investigations. At the Friday tutorial Dr S said at the start: 'Before we get on to today's case presentation and tutorial, let's hear the answer to the question we left [student name] to work on.'

These scenarios show how a simple technique redirects responsibility for learning to the learner and results in a bit of work in flexible time to work out the answer. The process is a little longer, but learners often feel satisfied when they have worked things out themselves and made a contribution to group activities.

This concept is known as an 'educational prescription', pioneered by David Sackett. A variant of the concept has the clinical teacher imposing a learning task on him or herself, agreeing to look something up and report back at the next meeting. This is excellent role modelling of a competent clinician who must manage information in order to keep up to date. These suggestions are summarised in Box 3.9.

One worrying trend is the increasing proportion of students who choose or have to work part time to afford to be a student. Some will exploit 'flexible' time to work during normal working hours. While this is not a sound idea, as it means they will miss daytime learning opportunities, so long as they attend important sessions and perform the 'flexible' tasks during evenings or on weekends, they can still learn, even if they feel worn out. Similar challenges face students with small children, as caring for children will often (should?) be the first priority.

Box 3.9 Tips for using flexible time

- Arrange for students to see more patients between formal teaching sessions. If asked, assign some that you think match the current learning objectives.
- Ask students to do library research on topics they raise so that they learn how to apply information resources in clinical care.
- Allow students choice about when to conduct tasks in their own 'flexible' time.
- Be aware that some students will have part-time jobs and family commitments. If possible, allow flexible time activities to fit around personal commitments.

Providing learning support materials

Learners learn best when provided with messages that are repeated and are in different, ideally complementary, formats. Clinical teachers should not necessarily go to enormous lengths to produce sets of notes for their students, but may well have lists of current references that are worth looking up, and know of textbooks not on the recommended list, but in the library, that have particularly good images, diagrams or text descriptions. Others may have developed brief notes, based on years of experience. These materials are often very useful for students, as they will reinforce, elaborate and triangulate important messages. Handouts based on slide presentations should be provided in the format where students can add notes beside individual slides. However, clinical teachers should ensure that the notes are current, and this takes some effort every year or two to add new materials and delete outdated materials.

Clinical teachers should avoid recommending that students buy additional texts that are not on the recommended list, even if they personally think other books are better. Students generally cannot afford to buy many textbooks and those they do buy date rapidly. If other books are worth reading, lobby the medical school to provide copies in the library. These suggestions are summarised in Box 3.10.

Box 3.10 Tips for providing additional learning materials

- Keep lists of current references relevant to particular topics students must cover.
- Strive to have libraries hold copies of good textbooks that elaborate knowledge and understanding.
- Current, brief summaries of your experience with complex topics (time permitting) can be helpful.
- Hand out, or place on the web, copies of your slide presentations.
- Regularly update the materials.
- Do not urge students to purchase textbooks not on the recommended list; instead, make recommendations to the course directors.

Small group process

Most clinical teaching involves a clinical teacher and a group of students, perhaps two to 10 in total. This requires clinical teachers to have some understanding of small group dynamics and how to manage small groups.

Scenario 3.20

Dr T met her new group of six students at 10 am for the first tutorial of the clinical rotation. She began by welcoming the students to the clinical rotation and to her ward in particular. She explained that this week she would present a case as a guide to what they would be expected to do in coming weeks, and proceeded with the case presentation. After 15 minutes she finished, asked if there were any questions and then asked individual students questions, explaining that this would help her sort out who knew their stuff.

Scenario 3.21

Dr U met his new group of six students at 10 am for the first tutorial of the clinical rotation. He began by welcoming the students to the clinical rotation and to his ward in particular. He gave a brief summary of his clinical qualifications and background, and told them about his wife and three children. He then asked each student to introduce themselves to each other and to him, and for each one he asked about their personal lives and how they viewed medicine as a career. By the time all had done this, the tutorial was over.

New groups of students need to introduce themselves to each other, but it is likely that medical students in a group already know each other, unless it is early in the academic year. It is wise to ask them if they know each other rather than assume that they do. Introductions are sound practice, and here the key party is the clinical teacher, who should explain a bit about him or herself. Including some personal stuff makes the teacher appear to be a person, not a machine, but it can be overdone. Students may not want to talk much about their personal lives, particularly in a group situation, so clinical teachers who want to know more about individual students might be better off arranging one-to-one meetings around clinical teaching issues. However, care needs to be taken to maintain the mostly professional relationship.

Is it acceptable for the first tutorial to spend more time on group process than on content? Absolutely! Establishing sound communication and trust will make things flow better in tutorials that follow, so anticipate the need to do this.

Box 3.11 Tips for managing small groups of learners

- Plan ahead and allow for a greater process than content focus in the first tutorial. Introduce yourself and include information about your life away from work.
- Have all members introduce themselves (or each other) to you.
- Regularly observe each group member and get to understand his or her personality.
- Work out the more dominant members of the group and discourage their dominance.
- Work out the more introverted members of the group and encourage their participation.
- Have the group appoint a different chair for each meeting (or week) and rotate the chair position to all members.

Continued

- Allow some social chat, but regularly return the focus of meetings to the task.
- Have some meetings away from the formal rooms, such as in a coffee shop over the road.

Small group management requires constant observation of all participants. Groups sometimes have a confident extrovert who will lead. Some will have an under confident introvert who will hide behind others. The latter can still participate actively in an intellectual sense, as the discussions are internal – monitor this by watching their eye contact and other non-verbal behaviour. If there is more than one overconfident extrovert, the group process can degenerate to a level of competition between them for air time and switching off by the others. Small group leaders need to monitor participation by all group members and try to see that all get equal access to the discussion and are able to ask their questions. Box 3.11 summarises some of these tips, but there are many good books on small group process (*see* Further reading).

Case presentations

Case presentations are a variation on small group process. They are a common format for both teaching and assessment, and their role in assessment will be discussed further in Chapter 5. Depending on how they are conducted, they can be either the most or the least interesting activities for medical students.

Scenario 3.22

Dr V was the registrar whose turn it was to present a case at the weekly departmental meeting. This was an anxious event for Dr V, because she was presenting to a mixed audience that included senior consultants, other registrars and junior hospital staff, and the current group of medical students, and she did not want to appear 'ignorant' in front of anyone! She had an overhead projector on which was a page of typed (font 12) notes that began with the patient's presenting complaint. This was a patient who had been referred from a district hospital for more specialised investigation at a time when the diagnosis was not clear, and turned out to have a very rare condition that many clinicians missed. Dr V proceeded to read her summary sequentially, going through the patient's presenting history and examination findings, the initial investigations and differential diagnoses, and to the final diagnosis. After 40 minutes she stopped and asked for questions.

Scenario 3.23

A student was taking his turn to present a case as all had to do this once during the clinical rotation. He put up an overhead slide with the patient's presenting symptoms. Before he could continue Dr W, the clinical teacher, said to the whole group: 'Thanks for that. Now, based on just that information, what kinds of problems are you thinking this patient might have?' The following discussion involved all the students. Several suggestions, some of them quite unlikely, were made, but Dr W did not comment. He then asked: 'What other questions would you like to ask? Your colleague presenting the case should know enough about the patient to answer them.' The case presentation continued, with regular pauses to question the audience about the themes and information synthesis.

I am sure that Scenario 3.22 is familiar to most readers. Several questions arise. For whom is such a meeting being run? Who is most likely to benefit? Is it aimed at continuing professional development for the senior consultants, a 'trial by ordeal' experience for the registrar who aspires to be a consultant, or a learning session for medical students? In many ways it is an anti-educational process, with an individual (the presenter) feeling under intense scrutiny and too many levels of learner in the audience for the needs of all to be addressed. The students probably learn very little, and indeed many in the audience will be squirming and hoping that they will not be asked a question in such an intimidating environment. The 'St Elsewhere's' phenomenon (blaming other, often lesser equipped, hospitals) is also commonly encountered in teaching hospitals, even though any objective analysis would indicate that difficult diagnoses are generally difficult to make, even in the best facilities.

In Scenario 3.23, the focus is clearly on learning and, in this case, on a particular level of learning – medical students. That might seem to be a luxury that many clinical teachers cannot afford, but it highlights the issue of tailoring case presentations to the needs of the target group. Making a case presentation meet the learning needs of more than one target group – say students and registrars – is more difficult. Ideally, students and registrars should have separate discussions, calibrated to the different levels of learning.

As a rule, if students are supposed to learn, the case presentations should be tailored to their needs. The practice of inviting them to big departmental 'grand rounds' and case presentations for registrars might be useful and interesting, but should be seen as additional, not core, activities. Some suggestions for facilitating case presentations are summarised in Box 3.12.

Box 3.12 Suggestions for facilitating case presentations

- Design the presentation to be primarily for medical students.
- Discourage long presentations with crowded overhead slides.
- Pause frequently to discuss the patient.
- Ask many questions and give few direct answers.
- Monitor small group function to maximise participation.
- Suggest 'homework' to follow up unanswered questions.

Dealing with academic performance and personal problems

For reasons that are not entirely clear, academic and personal problems are relatively common in medical students. Perhaps it is the length of the course, the high academic and community expectations, or the nature of the professional tasks. In any case, medical schools have to provide, or be able to refer to, a range of academic and personal support services, and clinical teachers may well be the first to detect any problems.

Diagnosing learning difficulties

Most students are academic high achievers, but it is a mistake to assume that none will have some form of learning disability. Most are reasonably high-order disabilities that might not impair the function of people in many walks of life, and are therefore hard to detect. Students admitted through widening access programmes may have more varied prior academic preparation and show a higher rate of special learning needs. Consider the following scenarios and try to work out what the problems might be.

Scenario 3.24

The multiple-choice question (MCQ) examination paper in the medical course included several extended matching questions (EMQs), a kind of MCQ that has up to 20 or so possible answers. Students are required to shade a small circle on a marking sheet that is computer scanned, but the form is different from previous MCQ marking sheets as there are one and a half rows of circles for each question. One student does very poorly on the EMQ section of the paper and fails the MCQ paper overall. An astute education officer checks the scoring sheet and finds that the student appears to have made an error in using the scoring sheet and, once the pattern is recognised, probably should have passed the paper.

Scenario 3.25

The students were required to complete an individual assignment, based on writing up a clinical case, worth 10% of the total score for the year. One of the clinical teachers who was marking the case study noticed that two assignments appeared to have a lot of words in common, almost as if one was copied directly from the other. This was reported to the senior academic staff of the school, who investigated the situation and found that these two students often worked together, and one was not good at reading and writing, even though he had done quite well academically in other assessment formats in maths and science subjects. The two students were called in to discuss an allegation of plagiarism.

Mild 'learning problems' that are commonly encountered include students with weaker skills in oral or written communication. Many medical students achieve very high academic scores in pre-medical school assessments on the basis of outstanding mathematic and scientific ability. Most of these will be 'all round' high achievers, but some will not be great readers or talkers. A few of the latter might have reading comprehension problems that impair their capacity to process large amounts of written information and to write coherent essays or case studies, even though their knowledge base might be sound. Some might also have problems organising information within their memories and in structuring information in written or verbal presentations in what most would regard as a logical manner. Such problems can be quite troubling for students, who may never before have been regarded as strugglers, but their assessment scores dive when they are primarily assessed on the bases of case studies and clinical presentations. The most subtle cases are usually high-achieving students studying in their first language, but these kinds of problems are also more common in students learning medicine in their second or third language, most commonly recent immigrant and international students.

The scenarios provide examples of two common forms of language and literacy problems. They are more commonly found in males and they can exist in medical students; the problems do not necessarily mean poor academic ability in many aspects of learning. In both scenarios, the student probably has some kind of reading and writing problem. In the first it is most obvious when having to read and understand a complex scoring form, and in the second it limits the ability to write original prose. Some students try to cover this up by asking friends for notes and other materials to copy, and may get detected as possible perpetrators of plagiarism.

The important issue is to recognise when a student might fall into the category of having some form of learning disability and referring them for assistance. Students with different language backgrounds and international students usually have specific support systems, but others may need an assessment by an educational psychologist and specific support to develop missing skills. Some tips for identifying and dealing with possible learning problems are listed in Box 3.13.

Box 3.13 Tips for identifying and dealing with possible learning problems

- Take note if students appear to have problems understanding number sequences and written notes or reports.
- Think of language and literacy problems if students appear to be copying information directly from their peers in assignments.
- Report any suspicions to senior school staff.

Diagnosing students with personal problems

Medical students may come from the upper end of the scale of academic ability and perhaps even socio-economic status, but they are otherwise normal human beings and can suffer the same kind of health problems as the rest of the community. Indeed, the medical profession is more prone to certain problems, such as alcohol and drug dependence and suicide risk, and these issues are relevant to medical students also.

Medical students are mostly young adults and school-leavers are still really adolescents when they start. They may not be certain of their sexuality, be prone to risk-taking behaviour typical of the age, and can suffer from the same range of physical and mental health problems as other adolescents and young adults. Many of the younger students may be living away from home for the first time and having to grapple with the increased independence that brings. Older students often have other pressures, such as families to support and mortgages to pay off. Many, regardless of their age, are slightly obsessional high achievers who are driven by success.

Scenario 3.26

The new term began with a group of apparently motivated students. However, after the first week one student stopped attending teaching sessions regularly. When he did attend he was almost always late. He stayed at the back of the group and rarely participated in discussions, appearing to be distracted. After three weeks and during another of his absences, the tutor, Dr X, asked where he was. The other students looked at each other nervously and one said: 'We're a bit worried about him too. He seems to have lost interest and we think there are big problems at home.'

Scenario 3.27

A student was one of a pair attached for a short placement in a rural community and was living in the old staff quarters building. She attended well and, apart from being a bit anxious, appeared to be normal. After a few days the other student came to the preceptor, Dr Y, and expressed concern about her colleague. She said that she noticed that the other student ate really large meals at night, but could be heard throwing up in the communal toilets later each night. Dr Y then realised that the student was also very thin.

The closer relationship between clinical teachers and students means that, sometimes for the first time, an experienced medical practitioner teacher sees each student very often and up close. This means that behaviours that may be missed in larger groups become more obvious. For example, poor attendance, sloppy dress standards and poor participation are more easily spotted. In rural placements students are more visible after hours, and personal problems that can be hidden by day often become evident.

Clinical teachers have to be prepared for the inevitability that some day they will encounter a student with a personal problem, and know how to manage that inevitability. They must be prepared to recognise that a problem might exist and do something about it; it is better to later find out that there is no serious problem than to have to deal with a suicide or admission to hospital that might have been preventable. They then must know what to do. This means letting someone in the medical school know – there are academics with responsibility for student issues in every medical school – either directly or through the local course coordinator within the health facility. If students will not agree to that, then referral to an appropriate person (say, a psychiatrist) might be necessary. Clinical teachers should *not* agree to personally manage a student with a personal problem, as this mixes the relationships and might impair one or both relationships. Tips for handling personal problems are listed in Box 3.14.

Box 3.14 Tips for identifying and helping students with personal problems

- Be aware that students can have personal problems.
- Consider personal problems if students attend poorly, seem very withdrawn or have unexpectedly poor assessment results.
- Never take on a student with personal problems as a patient.
- Know where to refer students for assistance.

Summary

This chapter has provided a series of case scenarios that illustrate selected practical clinical teaching skills, discussing their weaknesses and strengths, and presenting suggestions for improving the educational outcomes. The next chapter focuses on how to implement these clinical teaching skills in a range of clinical settings.

Further reading

- Chew-Graham C, Rogers A and Yassin N (2003) 'I wouldn't want it on my CV or their records': medical students' experiences of help-seeking for mental health problems. *Medical Education.* **37**(10): 873–80.
  Medical students who admit to having mental health problems may face barriers to later careers and so avoid seeking help.
- Givens JL and Tija J (2002) Depressed medical students' use of mental health services and barriers to use. *Academic Medicine.* **77**: 918–21.
  Research that suggests that depression in medical students is common, yet under-recognised.
- Newble D and Cannon R (2001) *A Handbook for Medical Teachers* (4e). Kluwer Academic Publishers, Dordrecht.
  Full of practical information about how to create teaching sessions – particularly relevant to more traditional forms of clinical teaching.

- Pendleton D *et al.* (1984) *The Consultation. An approach to teaching and learning.* Oxford University Press, Oxford.
  Perhaps the most widely referenced textbook on communication skills in medicine, and relevant beyond its primary care focus.
- Sayer M, De Saintonge MC, Evans D *et al.* (2002) Support for students with academic difficulties. *Medical Education.* **36**: 643–50.
  Research that demonstrates that academic failure among students is often not due to academic problems, some of which are able to be remediated.
- Whitman N (1990) *Creative Medical Teaching.* Department of Family and Preventive Medicine, University of Utah School of Medicine, Salt Lake City.
  Full of innovative and interesting teaching and learning strategies, including games and fun activities that are ideal as ice-breakers and learning enhancers, mostly designed for group learning.
- Whitman N and Schwenk TL (1997) *The Physician as Teacher* (2e). Whitman Associates, Salt Lake City.
  Simple and readable book about teaching in mostly inpatient clinical settings, with a US flavour.

Chapter 4

Teaching in common clinical settings

> For rigorous teachers seized my youth,
> And other its faith, and trimmed its fire,
> Showed me the high, white star of truth,
> There bade me gaze, and there aspire.
>
> Matthew Arnold, 1855

Introduction

This chapter presents scenarios that illustrate teaching encounters in a variety of commonly used clinical settings. Medical schools have to extend clinical experience and supervision experiences for their students to settings where students have not normally been present, and also have to consider 'smarter' ways of using the more traditional settings to provide adequate opportunities to learn how to be a medical practitioner in the near future. In particular, hospital-based clinical teachers need to think about how to include community and primary care as a setting in which students learn about hospital medicine. This is not really as revolutionary as it sounds, as more and more hospital medicine is being relocated to community care teams.

As with the last chapter, important issues are illustrated in short scenarios, all based on genuine events, in which readers are encouraged to identify any issues and reflect on their own teaching experiences. Once again, ask yourself some questions about each scenario.

1 What teaching and learning mechanisms were in operation?
2 How well would the learners have been motivated, engaged and able to learn?
3 Who got the most out of the encounter?
4 How could learning have been improved?

Inpatient teaching in hospital wards

Hospital wards in the large public teaching hospitals are perhaps the most traditional of all clinical settings used by medical schools. Here lies a concentration of interesting and complex problems from which students can learn a lot. The usual model is that students are attached in small groups to a 'unit', a 'firm' or whatever the clinical unit is called. This unit will include one or more consultants (honoraries or attendings), a specialist in training (registrar or resident), and recent medical graduates, perhaps in their first postgraduate year. The principle is that the learners, and here there are three levels of learner (four if consultants are included as learners!), work as a team that provides clinical care to a list of patients, follow or 'shadow' their more experienced colleagues and learn by watching and doing.

The quality of healthcare now depends on much more than the effort of a few individuals. Issues such as teamwork, clinical information management and communication skills have assumed much greater importance. Hence, clinical teaching needs to provide much more than the traditional issues of how to apply knowledge and skills. However, learning how to apply knowledge, skills and attitudes remains a very important aspect of any clinical teaching experience.

Core clinical teaching and learning

Large teaching hospitals are very busy places with patients moving through them quite quickly. Modern striving for efficiency requires their passage to be fast, unless there are unusual complications or greater than normal complexity. Many of the patients passing through have stories to tell, and signs to demonstrate, that provide ideal learning opportunities for medical students. The stories and signs are not always fascinating, but the majority of healthcare is about ordinary people with ordinary problems.

Scenario 4.1

The students arrived in the ward at 8.30 am and asked the registrar, Dr A, about patients admitted during the previous night. Dr A said that there were only three (what a relief, she said!) and that they were not very interesting. One was an elderly man with a slight stroke, another a middle-aged woman with pneumonia, and the third was an elderly woman with an exacerbation of heart failure. The students felt that they had seen enough of such problems already and went to the coffee shop to discuss their case presentations to be made later that week. Dr A was pleased to get on with her busy clinical duties.

Scenario 4.2

The group of students attached to medical unit 3 were each allocated a day and evening to be 'on call' to admit any new patients, while another was available for ward calls from the nursing staff. Each time the student was called, he or she would see the patient alone, take a history, conduct an examination, make an assessment of the patient's problems and write all this in the patient's record. The student would then ring the registrar (for admissions) or JHO (for ward calls) and present the patient, based on their findings, for discussion and feedback, sometimes before approving action, sometimes later. A student interacted with every admitted patient and therefore every patient was discussed with the group.

Medical students can probably not see too many patients. Even where they have seen many similar patients and problems, each patient presents a little differently and the encounter is stored as a script in memory, assisting later diagnostic processes (*see* diagnostic reasoning in Chapter 7).

Students learn more when they are participants in healthcare, with a role that is recognised as being useful. Students should interact with all consenting patients, with supervision, feedback, advice and opportunities to gain experience. Attaching students to patients, not firms or units, helps them see where their source of real learning is. Scenario 4.2 shows how students can learn from every single patient admitted for medical care.

The challenging clinical dilemmas

One of the reasons why teaching hospitals are regarded as great teaching environments is that they attract complex, rare and fascinating clinic cases. Clinicians in large teaching hospitals are often relatively expert in this kind of medicine and attract such patients from a substantial population base.

Scenario 4.3

The word got out that a woman with an 'amazing' breast tumour was in ward 5, bed 12, awaiting surgery the next day. For some reason she had presented late and therefore provided a rare opportunity for learners to feel a real and relatively advanced tumour. The unofficial advice from mentors was that all students should make the effort to examine her left breast. Group by group, students in all clinical years wandered up and joined what turned out to be a longish queue. When one particular group arrived, they saw about seven or eight students ahead of them, waiting near a bed that was curtained off. The patient was in her 40s and, as the curtains were opened between students, she appeared to be quite an attractive, but rather unhappy, person. Each student was in there for about two minutes, saying something like 'Sorry, is it OK if I check it too?' and getting out as fast as possible, looking almost embarrassed. None seemed to even attempt to connect emotionally with her. One of the junior nurses came by and said quietly to some of those in the queue: 'Why are you doing this to her? About 40 students have come through so far today and she was in tears after the last lot finished before lunch.' Some of the students felt ashamed, drifted away and never got to feel that particular tumour. Others stayed and felt the tumour, saying that the patient understood that they needed to learn.

Scenario 4.4

The endocrinology ward had 30 beds and the occupancy rate was at close to the usual 100%. There was the usual mix of patients with a range of conditions, primarily diabetes and thyroid disease, most of them either very difficult or very complex. One patient with diabetes was proving to be very difficult to manage and was found to have an insulinoma. The registrars and consultants were very excited as this was a relatively rare event. Discussions

Continued

in all the tutorials that week were dominated by this complex case and the students all saw the patient and researched the current diagnostic and management issues on Medline. That week, the other 29 patients were hardly involved in the students' teaching and learning activities.

One of the disadvantages of the common focus on fascinating cases is that students pay less attention to the kind of medical problems they are much more likely to have to deal with later. Further, they have a relatively narrow experience of normal human structure and function.

Scenario 4.3 is not so uncommon, although one would hope that the more recent focus on holistic care would allow students to see that queuing up for a quick prod of an advanced tumour with a terrible prognosis without acknowledging the emotional environment is unacceptable. It is being increasingly recognised that patients have rights too.

Scenario 4.4 is more common in more specialised hospitals, where it is sometimes difficult to find any patients with 'ordinary' conditions that are more relevant to the medical school curriculum. Higher complexity of patient problems is becoming much more common in teaching hospitals, and is very relevant to the learning needs of registrars and continuing professional needs of consultants, but less so to those of students.

In many respects the fascinating or very complex ends of the clinical spectrum are less valuable for medical student learning; they really need to focus on the more common conditions that they will need to deal with prior to postgraduate training. Students who master the more common issues may of course be stretched a little, but this should not be expected of the majority. Medical students will often have richer and more relevant learning experiences in smaller, district hospitals.

Access to academically bright teachers

Another advantage of a teaching hospital environment is that it is a site of training for specialists. Training registrars are often academically bright, highly motivated, driven by success, and approaching high-stakes examinations that could determine their future. Much of the medical student teaching in teaching hospitals is in the hands of the registrars, so surely exposure to these people is a positive influence on medical students!

Scenario 4.5

Others said how lucky this group of students was because their registrar, Dr B, was in advanced training and he really knew his stuff! He was also a bit of a slave driver, assigning students to patients, watching them from afar and then reading their case studies. He would get upset if a student spent less than two hours with a patient, did not record every possible positive and negative finding (particularly the latter), suggest a very long list of differential diagnoses, and then recommend ordering a long (and expensive) list of investigations. Many of the patients in his ward had renal problems. All students soon learned that the way to get good marks was to make it clear that they had seriously considered a condition called paroxysmal nocturnal haematuria, with all the associated symptoms, signs recorded negatively and the investigations for it proudly discussed, along with management options, even when this was a most unlikely possible diagnosis. However, none of the students knew what the condition was and none of the patients were ever discovered to have it. They worked out how to keep him happy but were not sure that they learned as much about a wide range of conditions as students in other groups.

Scenario 4.6

The hospital's best-known registrar was Dr C; he was tall, good looking and he took a strong interest in his students. He had passed his specialist exams and would soon be a consultant, and everybody knew he would be a professor one day – he was just so good at teaching! Students loved working in his ward, because he knew just about everything, often through clever memory-prompts that he either learned elsewhere or made up himself. He seemed to know 10 answers for every question, no matter how rare the condition, test or result – a real walking encyclopaedia! He was a particularly popular person when students needed to find out something. All they had to do was ask him and he would rattle off the relevant information in a flash – they rarely had to look in a textbook or go to the library. What's more, he was willing to pass his knowledge on to students, grilling them over and over until they could recite long lists of possible causes and investigations. Students in other groups often felt inferior to Dr C's!

These scenarios raise important educational questions. The first is: whose learning agenda is being dealt with here? Both registrars do not appear to be attuned to what the students need to know, but instead are following highly individual paths. Dr B appears to be obsessed with exotic differential diagnoses and Dr C with cramming knowledge into simple memorising tools. Both may at times be reasonable topics or approaches, but should not dominate the learning experiences of students who are at a lower level.

A second question relates to the debate about whether students need to first learn either a very comprehensive or a more focused approach to information gathering. Dr B clearly believes in ramming home a very comprehensive approach that is rarely used by experienced doctors, but clearly all do need to know it when confronted by unusual presentations (*see* diagnostic reasoning in Chapter 7). There is not necessarily a right answer to the debate, as both are needed, but there needs to be balance.

The third question relates to how much a clinical teacher should control the learning, compared to how much the students should be allowed to learn by discovery. Both Drs B and C demonstrate a rather didactic style that risks signalling to students that learning is not their own personal responsibility. Dr

C probably 'spoon feeds' too much, perhaps realising that memorising lists is of only limited and short-term help, as lists will change in different contexts and over time.

Teamwork

One of the more traditional views of healthcare has the doctor at the apex of a pyramidal system, playing the vital roles of knowledge expert and manager. The medical team in a hospital setting used to be a consultant, a registrar and junior medical officers, with some students as an appendage. This model has changed substantially to one where several people provide expertise in content knowledge, process management, leadership and communication. There are usually several doctors in the team, as well as several nurses, together with various combinations of pharmacists, physiotherapists, occupational therapists, speech therapists, psychologists and social workers. In addition, there are people who coordinate care from so many different players. In effect there are several overlapping teams of professional people involved in patient care. Medical students need to see this teamwork happening, participate in its function, and learn its value to patient care.

Scenario 4.7

Students were allocated a patient each, and allowed a few days to interview and examine the patient and then develop a case presentation for a tutorial discussion. As part of their presentation work-up they were required to speak with every health professional involved with the care of the patient and seek their views on the patient's management and prognosis. These health professionals were then invited to the tutorial to participate in the discussion.

Scenario 4.8

The hospital unit for the new rotation was managed differently to others the students had seen. Ward rounds were relatively brief and the students did not have to attend, although were encouraged to attend some rounds in ones or twos at the most. The rounds were very much 'business' rounds, where patient histories and examination findings were updated, primarily by the junior medical officers most involved in their care, with very little discussion. After the round, the medical team would be joined in an adjacent tutorial room by more nurses and the therapists and pharmacist most involved with the ward. Each patient was then presented to the broader team, and each person was asked to comment on the patient from their perspective. Decisions were made about further investigation, management or discharge, with reasons discussed. After the case conferences the registrar and students went around the ward again, explaining the outcome to the patients.

Medical students can, and should, learn from all health professionals involved in patient care. This has of course always happened to a certain extent, but the increasing contribution of more specialised knowledge and skills from a wide range of other professions means that medical students must learn about those contributions and how professionals combine to produce high-quality healthcare. Medical students do not need to acquire the content expertise of those other professionals, but do need to know how to arrange access to the expertise, as required.

This brings into focus inter-professional communication. Health professionals should work together harmoniously to produce commonly desired patient care outcomes, and therefore need to be able to communicate effectively and respectfully in order to achieve efficient collaboration. These skills can be role-modelled by clinical teachers and indeed the entire healthcare team.

Clinical information management

In this more complex world, where there are so many players and rapid development of technology, the management of clinical information is becoming crucial to healthcare and to the roles played by doctors.

Scenario 4.9

The unit had two new medical students starting and they met with the whole unit team early on Monday morning, just prior to the ward round. The consultant, Dr D, was an experienced and respected senior clinician who enjoyed teaching medical students. After the introductions he said to one of the students: 'You may as well start off on day one being part of the team. I would like you to be the scribe for the ward round today. Listen carefully and jot down the important points in the patients' records as we go.' The student had read a few patient records before, but had never written much in them, and was very nervous about this task. He did his best, but at the end of the round the consultant looked at what he had written. He commented that the student had written too much, probably not the most salient points, and that it was mostly illegible. However, with a smile, he said: 'Don't worry, the registrar has a great memory and will rewrite it.'

Scenario 4.10

The unit had two new medical students starting and they met with the whole unit team early on Monday morning, just prior to the ward round. The consultant, Dr E, was an experienced and respected senior clinician who enjoyed teaching medical students. After the introductions she said to one of the students: 'You may as well start off on day one being part of the team. I would like you to be the scribe for the ward round today. Have you done that before? No, well, we will show you what to do. Listen carefully to

---

Continued

what we say and we will together decide the salient information that we should record on the first patient.' This happened and the students took part in discussions about what was important to record. One of the JHOs wrote the information into the patient's record, then all read it and agreed that is was OK. Dr E then said: 'Now you do the writing, but we will still discuss what to write as a group and then check what you have done.' The ward round continued, with the student gaining confidence and needing less discussion by the end of the round. Dr E then looked at the records and said: 'Well done – I guess your writing is typical of we doctors. I can't wait to get a wireless system for our hand-held PCs to make this easier, but you have recorded the relevant information. Tomorrow, your colleague can do this, then after that we will get you both to take turns.'

Recording legible, relevant and meaningful clinical information, and interpreting it, are important skills that need to be taught and coached the same way as other clinical skills. It appears to be a simple task, yet it requires substantial clinical knowledge and a sound understanding of how healthcare works. It may well not be appropriate for novice clinical learners, but more so for senior medical students who have a better grasp of the underlying knowledge and skills required.

On the face of it, Dr D begins well, showing that he wants students to learn the skill of writing in patient records, and even boldly throws the student into the role for some experiential learning. However, Dr D omits some important steps. He does not check how much the student knows about this skill. He does not demonstrate the correct way either before or during the round. He then risks turning the student off by feedback that verges on mocking. Dr E went further by providing the necessary coaching and feedback. Her students would have felt more empowered and confident than would Dr D's.

Contributing to and understanding patient records is only one aspect of current information management. The written approach in the scenarios may not be around much longer, as laptops and hand-held computers will become small and agile enough to perform this role, so long as support systems, such as wireless networks, become widespread. The most useful role of such technology may well be the easy access it provides to a range of clinical support systems, such as drugs databases, patient results and even bedside literature searches relevant to patient care. These developments need to be discussed and, where present, demonstrated and their appropriate use role-modelled.

Private hospitals

The private sector is a substantial part of several national healthcare systems, with many people holding private health insurance. This means that there may be a substantial proportion of hospital care provided outside of the public hospitals. Clearly, these provide opportunities for medical students to learn from patients and healthcare professionals.

Scenario 4.11

The medical school had negotiated access for their students to the XYZ private hospital and had a signed memorandum of understanding. As part of the negotiations, the dean wrote to every visiting medical officer (VMO) at the hospital, explaining the need for students to attend the private hospital and the curriculum model, and had sought their permission for students to approach their patients to seek consent for participation in teaching. All but two out of the 70 or so VMOs returned signed agreements that they would allow this to happen and that they would discuss their patients with students at mutually agreed times. After a few weeks the students complained that they rarely saw the VMOs because they came at times when the students were either busy or not present. When contacted the VMOs complained that the students were 'lazy' and not prepared to wait for them, although many acknowledged that they tended to visit their patients at odd times, generally early (e.g. 6.30 am) or late (e.g. 7 pm) in the day, in slightly unpredictable schedules.

Scenario 4.12

The medical school had negotiated access for their students to the XYZ private hospital and had a signed memorandum of understanding. As part of the negotiations, the dean wrote to every visiting medical officer (VMO) at the hospital, explaining the need for students to attend the private hospital and the curriculum model, and had sought their permission for students to approach their patients to seek consent for participation in teaching. All but two out of the 70 or so VMOs returned signed agreements that they would allow this to happen and that they would discuss their patients with students at mutually agreed times. However, all players recognised that the VMOs had time constraints dominated by the demands of private practice and that they were most unlikely to be able to make a reliable contribution to fixed teaching sessions. Therefore, the medical school employed experienced clinicians to go to the private hospital at agreed times to conduct the formal teaching sessions. This time was protected from other demands (some were part-time practitioners due to family needs or other interests) and the teachers were given VMO status within the hospital so that they had access to the facilities and resources. The formal student teaching took place as arranged and students were also able to have intermittent contact with the VMOs about their specific patients.

Including private hospitals in medical school teaching can be difficult. How well it works is clearly related to the structure of the local healthcare system. In some countries, public and private are separate systems, but many doctors work across both and are willing to teach in both. Private hospitals are also keen to become teaching sites for medical nursing and other health professional students, as this assists with accreditation of the hospital, adds interest to the professional lives of current staff members, and helps recruit future professional staff members. They are more likely than the public system to require formal agreements covering teaching, access to patients and facilities, and professional indemnity and insurance issues, although the public sector is becoming more inclined to also require that degree of formality.

There are, however, substantial differences to teaching in public hospitals. Private hospitals generally do not have in-house medical officers, except in high-dependency areas such as intensive care and coronary care units. Patients in wards are cared for by nursing staff, with private medical practitioners visiting briefly at times of largely their own convenience. The workload is also more surgically oriented, so the patient case-mix is quite different to large public hospitals. Therefore, students should be in the private sector for only a part, not the whole, of their learning experience. Patient consent also has to be more explicit, as does the consent of the VMOs, as the environment is more 'customer focused'.

However, if these structural issues can be addressed, students can learn a lot from patients in private hospitals, as their problems are often more suited to a medical school curriculum. The patients often have simpler medical problems and, in the surgical area, are often more healthy than the average, complex public hospital patient. Hence students, with guidance, can gain valuable experience of relatively healthy patients and a wider experience of normal clinical examination findings, and also wider experience in communication skills with different kinds of patients.

The medical school cannot, however, rely on VMOs to provide the formal teaching. Instead, individuals who can devote the time should be appointed and paid to be the main clinical teachers, with the VMOs providing valuable contributions when contacted by students about specific issues.

Operating theatres

The operating theatre is another traditional site of clinical teaching. Junior medical students often feel like it is 'the real thing' when they scrub, gown and glove up and enter the temple of surgery. Here they can observe teams in action, performing sometimes amazing things that make a big or immediate difference to health and life. Some surgeons are very keen to get students involved by having them assist in procedures, as they remember how excited they were by doing that many years ago.

Assisting in the operating theatre

On the face of it, assisting in theatre offers wonderful opportunities to be part of, and learn from, real surgical care.

Scenario 4.13

'How would you like to wash your hands and assist me with this operation?' said the consultant surgeon, Dr F. 'That way you will see living anatomy and pathology!' The medical student was just entering her first clinical year and was thrilled to say yes to this amazing invitation. However, she was not sure what to do in an operating theatre. Even though she had observed this several times, nobody has really shown her how to conduct a surgical scrub or put on a gown and gloves aseptically. She was therefore slower than the experienced surgeons and registrars, and made it into the theatre late. By then the patient was draped and the scrub nurse, registrar and intern were already surrounding the anaesthetised patient. Dr F loudly called out: 'Where is that student – come on around here – *no*, do not touch that drape or else the nurse will eat you! Come in here – closer, closer, you want to see what we are doing – *no*, not that close, don't touch his back. Look over here – see we are in the abdomen and the appendix is just under here. You probably can't see it as we arc into keyhole surgery now – patients do not want big scars. How about you help by holding this retractor? Good, I will place it in the right place and you just pull on it gently – *no*, too hard, it slipped', etc.

Scenario 4.14

The orthopaedic surgeon, Dr G, let it be known that every Thursday morning he was keen to have a student scrub up and be a second assistant for his list. Early in each rotation some students were keen to do this as they could practise the techniques of scrubbing, gowning and gloving, and were able to get very close to the action. However, they soon learned that some operations were less interesting than others. While they were quite keen to be there for arthroscopies, as they could watch a screen and see the inside of joints and the procedures were quite short, they did not enjoy assisting at total hip replacements, as it became clear that Dr G needed somebody of a certain height to support and rotate a limb for a substantial period of time at a vital stage of the procedure. The students soon learned to check what was on the list the previous day and make themselves scarce until the difficult procedures were over. Dr G became quite frustrated and complained to the medical school that the students were poorly motivated and would never be much good at orthopaedics.

There are some pitfalls in assisting surgeons in operating theatres. While the practice in sterile techniques is important and valuable, assisting well requires reasonable depth of knowledge about the condition and the technique, assets that few medical students will possess. Surgeons are generally enjoying what they do and are so engrossed that they do not notice time. They often can no longer see things from the point of view of a novice, who cannot follow the procedure and gets bored. Also, some assisting tasks really need a piece of equipment (robot arms are becoming more common!), not a human, and students should not be used (abused?) inappropriately.

In Scenario 4.13 the student was not really enjoying the experience, as she was not really able to see anything and constantly felt as if she was doing the wrong thing. This closes minds to learning. More experienced students often try to avoid assisting during the day when operating theatres are full of people, preferring to do so after hours when they might get closer to the action and get to do something useful.

These problems arise when surgeons regard operating theatre experience as an end, rather than as a means to an end. Medical students do not need to know much detail about procedures and techniques, but do need to understand principles of surgical management. The challenge for clinicians is to find ways of making assisting more valuable and more relevant to the medical school curriculum.

Longitudinal experiences of surgical management

One way of making operating theatre experiences more relevant to students is to make them just a part of the overall clinical experience with particular patients. Students really should see and be part of the surgical management of patients they are studying, and need to see less of procedures on patients they know little about.

Scenario 4.15

It was 10 pm on a Thursday night and a final-year student had followed a patient from initial presentation at around 5 pm, through admission to the ward, and now to the operating theatre, where he was asked by the registrar, Dr H, if he would like to assist with the appendectomy. He readily agreed, although was surprised by how long the wait was until the theatre and team were available. He was by now quite experienced in scrubbing, gloving and gowning and was soon standing opposite Dr H, acting as the only medical assistant – the consultant on call was happy not to be present unless needed for a complication and the JHO was busy with other admissions. The student was close enough to get an excellent look at living anatomy, as well as a slightly hot appendix, and enjoyed the experience immensely. The procedure went well and before long the appendix was removed, and the peritoneum was closed. Dr H's beeper then sounded an urgent tone. The scout nurse rang switchboard and conveyed the message that Dr G was urgently required by the JHO in one of the wards. Dr H suggested that the student finish closing the wound as she should attend to the urgent call now that 'the difficult stuff' was over.

Scenario 4.16

The big case on the next day's list was a 47-year-old man for resection of an early colonic cancer that was picked up on colonoscopy following a presentation with PR bleeding. The student knew that if she were to be allowed by the surgeon, Dr I, to get a close view of the anatomy and the procedure, she would have to interview and examine the patient that afternoon. She spent an hour with the patient and his family, asking them about his symptoms and signs, exploring his family history and discussing the impact of the diagnosis on the family. The next day the student was allowed to be second assistant and was close to the action. She maintained close contact during the post-operative period until discharge, and came to know the patient and his family quite well.

Both of these scenarios demonstrate how assisting in an operating theatre is an important part of the continuity of care experience of a medical student. Students can learn a lot after hours, when their assistance can even be very helpful. Dr H should of course not be leaving a student to complete the wound closure alone, as that demonstrates a mismatch of experience and responsibility. It also highlights a potential professional indemnity problem if things go wrong, as students have rights to be supervised and the registrar carries the professional indemnity risk. Back to the positives, both scenarios show how students can link components of medical care experienced by their patients, and learn from active rather than passive involvement. In Scenario 4.16, the positive contact with the patient and the family also sets up the possibility of even longer-term contact (*see* utilising primary care, p. 73).

Same-day services

The traditional academic teaching hospital has undergone substantial transformation during the last 20 years, as improvements in diagnostic technology and processes reduce the length of time and even the need for admission to hospital. The technology and process of clinical management have also developed substantially, resulting in a shorter average length of stay for those patients who are admitted to hospital. As a result, the number of 24-hour hospital beds has decreased, and a new form of hospital has emerged within or attached to the 24-hour facilities. These are the same-day services, where patients arrive at around 7 am, have investigative or treatment procedures, often under general or regional anaesthesia, and then go home by 4 pm to the care of their families. Some same-day services are free-standing, that is, not associated with hospitals.

Same-day services are often very efficient and they can be responsible for about half of the clinical activity in modern teaching hospitals, and some community hospital facilities provide only same-day services. Each year sees an increase in the number and range of clinical services that can be provided in same-day service facilities. Clearly, these facilities are too large to leave them out of clinical training for medical students.

Scenario 4.17

The student was rostered to attend the same-day gynaecology procedures list to observe some laparoscopies. She arrived at the appointed time, 8.30 am, with the gynaecologist, Dr J. They changed and went through to the procedures room, where the first patient was waiting for them under a light general anaesthetic. Each procedure was performed efficiently and the student was able to look down the laparoscope several times and see what female pelvic organs really looked like, and this was very satisfying. At the end of the list, Dr J went off to a clinic and the student went to a tutorial with the rest of her group, itching to tell the others about the pathology she saw.

Scenario 4.18

The student was rostered to attend the same-day gynaecology procedures list to learn how pathology matched clinical symptoms and signs. She arrived at 7 am, well before the gynaecologist, Dr K, and participated in the admission clerking of all patients on the list. She was able to interview all of them and to examine most of them abdominally, and explained to them that she would be present for their procedures. When Dr K arrived at 8.30 am, she went with him to the procedures room, where the first patient was waiting for them under a light GA. Each procedure was performed efficiently and the student was able to look down the laparoscope several times and see what female pelvic organs really looked like, and this was very satisfying. At the end of the list, Dr K went off to a clinic and the student went to a tutorial with the rest of her group, itching to tell the others about the pathology she saw, but they agreed to meet at 3 pm in the post-procedures room to jointly explain to each patient what they saw and what would happen next.

These scenarios show that same-day services offer rich learning opportunities if clinical teachers and students work out how to work within their efficient schedules. They allow students to follow patients through an episode of healthcare, to see the experience from the patients' perspective, and to see several procedures in a relatively short period of time. As with surgical patients in private hospitals, most same-day service patients are relatively healthy, and therefore offer many opportunities for medical students to practise communication, information gathering and examination skills, as well as opportunities to match pathology with clinical impressions, which will facilitate the learning of diagnostic reasoning.

Hospital outpatient clinics

Outpatient or ambulatory clinics have always had a role in medical school teaching, but their role has recently become more prominent, as changes to hospital function have reduced the availability of inpatients for teaching and learning. Hospital clinics are usually very busy places. Patients often wait a considerable time for the appointment; and some fail to attend. Some forget because the lead-time is so long, others have left town, improved or died. In response, clinics are often overbooked on the assumption that some will not show, rather like airlines do for scheduled flights. The result of this somewhat chaotic, inefficient system can be a somewhat chaotic, inefficient clinic, where there may be extreme pressure of work or unexpected gaps. Fitting teaching into this chaos is becoming more difficult. Teaching well in primary care settings probably slows service delivery by 25–30%, and while there are no similar figures for hospital clinics, the impact of teaching on service delivery is likely to be similar.

The use of hospital clinics is also changing. With the increased need to assess patients for the increasingly specialised, high-technology care options becoming available, greater emphasis is placed on referring patients back to the referring agency (usually primary care) once the more complex issues have been dealt with. As a result, patients are seen less often and that follow-up more often takes place in the referring setting.

Scenario 4.19

Two students have been scheduled to attend an outpatient clinic with a consultant, Dr L, with the objective of seeing patients with chronic diseases as they attend for follow-up a few weeks after discharge from a ward. The clinic is very busy, with about 60 patients booked over three hours to see either Dr L or the registrar, Dr M. As a rule, the workload is divided evenly between them. The students arrive at the appointed time and are allocated one each to the clinic rooms. However, they have not seen the patients before (they were in another term when these patients were inpatients) and the pressure of seeing 10 patients an hour means that they mostly just sit and listen to the doctors take a brief updating history and check on results from the inpatient episode, ensuring there are no loose ends.

Scenario 4.20

Two students have been scheduled to attend an outpatient clinic with a consultant, Dr N, with the objective of seeing patients with chronic diseases as they attend for follow-up a few weeks after discharge from a ward. The clinic is very busy, with about 60 patients booked over three hours to see either Dr N or the registrar, Dr O. As a rule, the workload is divided evenly between them. The students arrive at the appointed time to find that Dr N is running late and Dr O has had an urgent call to the wards. She apologises for leaving the students, but says: 'How about you help out? It is all really straightforward. All you have to do is ask them if they are now OK and check on results in the file from their admission, making sure there are no loose ends. If you have any problems, just get them to wait until I come back, otherwise just book them in again in a month and I will catch up.' The students work alone for almost an hour, finding the work relatively easy, and feeling like real doctors.

Scenario 4.21

Two students have been scheduled to attend an outpatient clinic with a consultant, Dr P, with the objective of seeing patients with chronic diseases as they attend for follow-up a few weeks after discharge from a ward. The clinic is very busy, with about 60 patients booked over three hours to see either Dr P or the registrar, Dr Q. The students are asked to arrive about an hour early to start off seeing two to three patients alone. These patients have been preselected on the basis of their clinical information and have been asked to come early and see a student first. The students each take a room and during the hour see these patients, taking a history, conducting a brief examination, checking on results of any clinical investigations, and trying to identify the issues to be dealt with today. When Drs P and Q arrive, the students briefly present their patients to one of them and they jointly identify learning issues relevant to the curriculum. This takes about an hour, after which the students go to the library to look up issues relevant to the patients, ready to meet with Drs P and Q at the end of the clinic for a more detailed discussion. Meanwhile, Drs P and Q get on with the service part of their clinics.

The traditional model of having students just observe (Scenario 4.19) is very inefficient for learning, although can be justified for a short while so that students become oriented to the function of a busy clinic. However, overuse results in yawning students losing motivation and busy clinicians who feel that students are slowing them down.

The solution probably lies in applying principles that by now should be familiar. Work out exactly what the students should achieve and what they should do to achieve it. Create a model of involving students in a way that minimises disruption to the service part of a clinic, but frees them to talk to and examine patients, read patient records, track down results and correspondence, and be a part of the healthcare team.

Scenario 4.20 shows one of the weaknesses of trying to teach in busy clinics with a shortage of medical staff. Medical students should be involved in a way that matches their learning needs, rights and responsibilities, and cannot be expected to play the role of a registrar, or even a junior medical officer, when supervisors are too busy to perform clinical work. The students may well make the right decisions, but have no legal status to work without supervision and support. Patients also have the right to be seen by a competent practitioner, even though a student may be a participant. If an error is made, the student may well feel dreadful, but the legal risk falls on the clinical teacher who failed to supervise properly.

Scenario 4.21 shows how time management through the organisation of a busy clinic can be changed to minimise disruption of service delivery. It probably takes a bit of time to establish and fine-tune, but once this is achieved, students can learn from patients and clinical teachers and be part of the team. The clinical teachers supervise as part of their service role rather than take time out to teach formally.

Utilising primary care

Another result of the increased efficiency of hospitals and same-day services is that more of the care has been moved from the hospital to the primary care sector. Many patients now have their diagnostic work-ups almost entirely in the community, prior to an admission to a hospital or same-day service. Similarly, most patients are discharged as soon as they are well and can be cared for in the community. While most patients prefer not to be in hospital for long, this drive for efficiency requires much more sophisticated community and primary care arrangements to cope with the additional work. Clearly, these arrangements provide opportunities for medical students to participate in healthcare and to learn both normal and abnormal human structure and function.

Scenario 4.22

The student had just completed an eight-week term in paediatrics at the teaching hospital and was now in week one of a four-week general practice attachment. The general practice was able to give him a rich clinical experience, allowing him to see patients initially alone, and then with an experienced general practitioner (GP), Dr R. The workload was diverse, and he enjoyed the variety. He even saw several children, sometimes for simple things like vaccinations, sometimes for management of asthma and diabetes. One of these – a 10-year-old, poorly controlled insulin-dependent diabetic boy – had recently been in hospital following a hypo and the student had had brief contact with him then. He found out from Dr R a lot of information that might have been useful during the admission, and he also thought of questions that he would like to ask the paediatricians he finished with last week, but they were now busy with another group.

Scenario 4.23

The student was in an eight-week term in paediatrics, primarily at the teaching hospital. Like all students, she was also attached to a general practice for part of every week of the clinical years. The practice encouraged her to be involved with as many of their consultations with children as possible, allowing her to see patients initially alone, and then with an experienced GP. She saw several children, sometimes for simple things like vaccinations, sometimes for management of asthma and diabetes. One of these – a 10-year-old, poorly controlled insulin-dependent diabetic boy – was having a lot of hypos. She asked his supervising GP, Dr S, why achieving compliance was so difficult, and also asked one of the hospital paediatricians the same question. She found out from Dr S a lot of background information about the boy and his family that was contributing to the problem, and went into the details of the insulin regime with the paediatrician, Dr T, and the diabetes educator. The student was able to see childhood diabetes from the perspectives of the patient, the family, the GP

Continued

and the specialist service, and even felt she had contributed to all parties gaining a better understanding of this particular case.

Scenario 4.24

The patient was ready for discharge after a brief admission for a series of complex investigations, and some of the results would not be available for a few days. A student took part in the discharge planning process, speaking with the patient when follow-up appointments were made with the patient's GP. The student arranged to be resent for this appointment through both obtaining the patient's permission and ringing the GP, Dr U, to arrange the appointment. At that follow-up visit, the student was able to contribute to Dr U's knowledge about what happened in hospital, be involved with explaining the results to the patient, and contribute to planning further management.

Scenario 4.25

The patient was ready for discharge after a brief admission for a series of complex investigations, and some of the results would not be available for a few days. A student took part in the discharge planning process, speaking with the patient when follow-up appointments were made at the specialist clinic in two weeks' time. The student arranged to visit the patient at home the next week to make an assessment of his progress, and arranged a time to speak to the patient's GP, Dr V, about his broader healthcare issues. The student then attended the follow-up appointment with Dr V, where she could speak knowledgeably about the patient's progress and contribute to the discussion about his future management.

Scenario 4.26

The elderly patient with recently diagnosed diabetes was to be discharged back to the care of her daughter, with a clinic appointment in four weeks' time. In the meantime, a community nurse was to visit each week to check that the daughter was managing the taking of blood sugar levels and dietary requirements. The student contacted the community nursing service to find out when these visits were to be made and arranged to attend them. At the follow-up clinic appointment four weeks later, the student was able to contribute knowledgeably about the patient's progress since admission.

Scenarios 4.22 to 4.26 illustrate how participation of students across the primary/secondary care 'divide' can facilitate deeper learning and, indeed, perhaps even contribute to improved care. Communication between primary and secondary care levels is often not as good as it should be, and involving students in a 'continuity' experience can both improve communication around specific patients and provide students with more information about patients they are studying. In both hospital and primary care settings the learning will often come from non-medical health professionals, and of course from patients, who can contribute their own unique perspective on what it is like to be the object of complex healthcare. A simple principle is to attach students to patients rather than individual clinical teachers or medical units, as patients are their prime source of learning. Clinical teachers are in both hospital and non-hospital settings and should work together to achieve the desired student learning outcomes.

Concurrent teaching and learning at multiple sites

As clinical education moves out of the large traditional teaching hospitals, medical schools quite often connect groups of students by either telephone or video conference. The two most often cited advantages are that it ensures that students at different sites are exposed to the same core teaching, and that it is more efficient than running each session several times (once at each site). With increasing moves to establish clinical teaching and learning in rural and remote settings, students and clinical teachers could be discussing clinical cases dozens of miles from each other, presented by students at any of the sites.

Scenario 4.27

There were 18 students and a clinical teacher (Dr W) at the main teaching hospital, with two groups of four connected in by telephone conference from two district hospitals, both of which were fifty miles away. One student in the larger group was presenting a clinical case for discussion, showing overhead transparencies summarising the key issues of history, examination and investigation findings. The discussion at the main site was quite animated with good participation from other students, but the students at the remote site did not have the transparencies and could not hear all of the discussion at the main site.

This is not an uncommon scenario. The students at the main site may have a reasonable educational experience, but those at the remote sites will be bored stiff as they cannot really participate. If such conditions continued over a series of tutorials, the students at the remote sites would almost certainly cease to attend regularly. Such behaviour would not necessarily signal poor motivation or learning, but rather that they had found a better way to learn what was necessary, perhaps alone or with other local students.

Facilitation of this kind of dispersed small group requires additional skills to those mentioned previously under small group process skills (*see* p. 48). The clinical teacher must take a very active role, making sure that the technology is working at all sites. Students should sit around a multi-directional microphone and speak clearly, one at a time. Students at remote sites should be regularly asked to comment as a check on their ability to hear and react to the presented material. Any presentations should be provided at all sites, either by emailing them as an attachment or faxing them. There should always be a back-up plan for when things go wrong. Should a technical glitch occur (and it will from time to time!), it may be better to disconnect remote sites and focus on local students for the moment, and arrange another time to repeat the session for the remote students. For video conferences, be aware that patterned, brightly coloured clothing and gestures can be hard to see in low mega-pixel images, and that drawings on white boards, particularly using several different coloured pens, transmit poorly with commonly available technology. These additional issues are summarised in Boxes 4.1 and 4.2.

Box 4.1 Multi-site tutorial facilitation

- Check that all sites are connected and the technology works.
- Email or fax presentations to all sites.
- Students should sit around multi-directional microphones.
- Everyone should speak clearly and one at a time.
- Regularly ask remote students questions and give them opportunities to comment.

Box 4.2 Additional issues relevant to video conference facilitation

- Wear clothes with solid colours, not patterns.
- Minimise movement.
- Do not transmit slides and images through the main camera: use document cameras and post or email slide presentations for local viewing.
- When drawing on whiteboards at the main site, make diagrams large and use strongly contrasting colours.

Making the most of any clinical setting

The scenarios in this chapter show that it is indeed possible to place students in a wide range of clinical settings, including the more recently emerging clinical services that do not keep patients for as long as previous models and so make patients less easily accessible to medical students. Further, community and primary care settings can provide learning experiences relevant to secondary and tertiary care medicine.

Box 4.3 Optimising learning in clinical settings

- Organisation and time management are essential.
- Link experiences to the curriculum and learning objectives.
- Ensure students learn what is normal as well as the abnormal.
- Focus on the strengths of particular clinical settings.
- Find students a useful role in the healthcare system.
- Attach students to patients to follow their healthcare journey.
- Involve a wide range of health professionals.
- Role-model professional teamwork.
- Guide students to cross health system compartments.
- Engage community and primary care.

The strategies that enable efficient use of patients and clinical settings are summarised in Box 4.3. Clinical teaching needs careful planning, as it does not just happen in a busy clinical service. The service either has to be organised around teaching, or teaching around the service, although a combination of the two is a likely and pragmatic outcome. Student activities within clinical settings must be linked to the curriculum and learning objectives, focusing in particular on what the particular clinical setting can offer. Students learn more when they have a defined role in the system, so long as it is at the appropriate level for their experience. Include all members of the healthcare team in the student experience and demonstrate effective teamwork that delivers better patient outcomes. Deliberately place students in both primary and secondary care settings as the two are becoming increasingly interconnected, and have them follow patients to and from different components of the healthcare system.

Summary

This chapter has used clinical teaching scenarios to assist readers to explore ways of extracting the most educational benefit from a range of clinical settings that can support teaching and learning, including newer clinical settings that are replacing or complementing the more traditional teaching hospital. Medical students can, and almost certainly should, be placed in a diverse range of clinical settings in order to achieve the learning objectives of current medical courses. The next chapter examines how clinical teachers in a wide range of clinical settings can make important contributions to the assessment of how well those learning objectives are achieved.

Further reading

- Irby DM (1995) Teaching and learning in ambulatory care settings: a thematic review of the literature. *Academic Medicine*. **70**: 898–909.
  A review of the evidence about what works best for teaching outside of traditional hospital settings. Although 10 years old, it is still worth reading, and it is of course relevant to teaching in hospitals too.

- Wallace P, Berlin A, Murray E *et al.* (2001) CeMENT: evaluation of a regional development programme integrating hospital and general practice clinical teaching for medical undergraduates. *Medical Education.* **35**: 160–6.
  Research showing that teaching in general practice can augment traditional hospital-based learning of core clinical skills.

Chapter 5

Determining whether or not learners have achieved the desired standard

The unexamined life is not worth living.
Plato, *c.*428–348 BC

Introduction

Medical schools believe that they have very simple needs of their clinical teachers in student assessment. They mostly want to know how well students are performing, so that they can be graded. Also, if students are not performing to a satisfactory standard, they like to know in broad terms what the problem might be, so that remediation can be offered.

This is a rather simplistic view, based on the widely held belief that all medical students are bright and should be able to do well. This is of course not necessarily true (otherwise, would we need formal assessment?), as medical courses are long and occur at an important time in the personal development of young adults. While at the beginning motivation and academic performance is generally high, by the more senior years some students may lose motivation, have personal or family problems, become ill, or be found to have a subtle learning problem. It is not uncommon for some students to struggle, even after successful completion of prior degrees and/or earlier years of medical courses. Therefore clinical teachers should know enough about assessment practices to be able to make fair and reasonable assessment decisions and to work out students' weaknesses.

Assessment in medical education is a huge topic, but clinical teachers do not need to become proficient in assessment theory, but rather proficient in making accurate judgements of how well students are performing. This chapter provides a practical approach to assessing learners, again using scenarios to prompt reflection, and focuses on assessment within clinical settings, where clinical teachers will be most likely to become involved in assessment of medical students. Chapter 8 provides a more theoretical approach to understanding assessment practices, aimed at clinical teachers who become more involved in high-stakes assessment or join assessment committees.

The assessment role of clinical teachers

Clinical teachers often feel uncomfortable when they are asked to assess the learners in their care. The nature of clinical supervision has teachers and learners seeing a lot of each other, sharing bonding experiences around interesting or exciting patient cases, and attending common medical social events. It should not be surprising that a common result is mutual respect and liking as junior and senior colleagues. Senior colleagues find it hard to criticise their junior colleagues. Many teachers enjoy helping their students to learn in an *ad hoc* manner from patients under their care, free of the constraints of assessments where they must make a judgement about eligibility to proceed to the next level. Indeed, many clinicians regard assessment as the 'enemy' of sound teaching practice, as students tend to focus on what is being assessed rather than what they might really need to learn.

However, assessment is an integral part of teaching and learning and must be planned and implemented as part of curriculum planning and implementation. The most important purpose of assessment is to assist learners to improve and to meet the required standards. Good teachers assess their learners more or less continuously, even if these assessments are not formal and decision making. Further, assessment practices, if designed well, should reinforce student learning of the intended curriculum. Learners like to receive feedback on their performance, so long as it is provided in a constructive way. Therefore, the assessment role should be seen as part of a constructive relationship between clinical teachers and their students.

Scenario 5.1

Dr A had agreed to be an examiner in the final clinical exam for the clinical rotation. She was observing students perform a physical examination on a real patient, Mr G, who had stable signs of chronic liver disease, completing a checklist and a rating scale for each student. The first four students performed adequately, indeed one very well, but the fifth started off wrongly and could not recover, and performed very poorly. Dr A was not at all surprised, as this student had been in her group for some of the rotation and he had performed poorly on every occasion. She had heard that he had family problems, limiting his attendance, and she wondered how much she should take this into consideration in scoring this examination.

Timing is everything

One of the key issues in blending teaching and assessing roles is to recognise that both are permanent roles, but that at certain times one may predominate. In Scenario 5.1, the clinical teacher may have confused the roles twice. The first time was weeks ago, when she recognised that this student was having problems, and did not act. If her judgement at that time was correct, she should have looked into the situation, referred the student to the proper place for advice, and offered additional teaching or coaching. At that time her main role was to help him learn, not make a dispassionate assessment of his ability.

The second time was during the examination, when it was not her role to consider adjusting scores because of the student's problems. At that time her main role was to make an objective assessment. If the student fails, others have the role of exploring the problem and developing a remediation programme to ensure he meets the required standard.

Formative and summative assessment

Clinical teachers are likely to contribute to two forms of assessment. The first is formative assessment, where learners are given feedback on their performance so that they become aware of their strengths and weaknesses, take action to correct any deficiencies, and continue to develop. Ideally, this is a friendly, open and confidential process that has no direct bearing on results, although some medical schools make it mandatory to participate in formative assessment. Students will be more comfortable participating in formative assessment if they know that it cannot be 'used against' them.

The second form of assessment is summative assessment, where the results contribute to a decision to pass or fail individual students, although should also provide feedback. Students have great difficulty regarding this as friendly and open, and can become quite stressed about it. Many clinical teachers will also find this role to be stressful, as they might make a decision that does not sit comfortably with their prior knowledge of the students. In the worst case scenario, they might have to contribute to a decision that might adversely affect a student's score or, less likely, inappropriately inflate the student's score.

Both roles are important, but the formative assessment role is the more important, and probably perennial, assessment role. More or less every assessment during clinical rotations should be used to provide feedback and constructive advice. If this is done well, students should enter examinations without major unresolved performance problems, and be able to pass comfortably. In most medical courses students are very dependent on their clinical teachers for formative assessment, as they are the most likely to observe them interact several times with patients and other health professionals, prior to the decision day. If the clinical teachers do not provide regular formative assessment, perhaps nobody will.

Scenario 5.2

Dr B had spent three to four hours each week with a group of six students and had come to know them well. He had observed each of them in several patient encounters, observed their interaction with other health professionals, discussed the list of core topics (plus a few extras) with them, asked them many questions and debated the answers, and chatted with them about medical life in the nearby coffee shop. He felt that he knew quite well their individual strengths and weaknesses. He had filled out several assessment rating forms for them, and given all of them quite high ratings as he felt they were performing well. He had also been asked to participate as an examiner in the forthcoming end of rotation examination, in which he may well have had to judge performance of some of these students in a clinical case.

Juggling hats

Students must receive fair and accurate assessment of their performance in both formative and summative assessment. Clinical teachers and students need to be comfortable with these roles. If the teacher–student relationship is strong, students will often accept summative assessment results better from people they know and trust. The nature of the relationship should be discussed early in a clinical rotation, using words like those given in Box 5.1. This is a form of verbal contract about duty of care that is implicit in clinical teaching, but perhaps should be explicit, and involve the students, as it makes clear to all the constructive nature of the relationship, but defines its limits.

Box 5.1 The clinical teacher – student duty of care

I am here to help you learn to become sound clinicians, based on all that knowledge you have acquired in the course. My guarantee to you is that I will do my best to help you achieve the expected standards. This means that I will watch carefully what each of you is doing. Where you do well, I will say so and explain how. Where I think you could do better, I will also explain how and help you improve. In return, I expect each of you to attend regularly, both for the tutorials and to see patients to practise your clinical skills, and to seek help if you are uncertain. During the rotation, my primary duty is to you and your learning.

  At the end of this rotation you will have to pass an assessment process and it is possible you will meet me there as an examiner. My role there is different, as my primary duty is to the medical school. I will still want you to do well, but I will have to judge objectively the performance of all students I assess there against the standards required by the medical school of your year group. If you have difficulties there I can provide feedback, but cannot alter the score. However, if we work well together during the rotation you should not have difficulties in the final assessment.

During assessment activities, clinical teachers should clearly understand (and identify to students, if it is not obvious) when the formative hat is being replaced by a summative hat. It may also be wise for clinical teachers not to assess summatively students whom they feel they know well. It is often standard practice in schools where there are logical ways of dividing students into groups based on different clinical teaching institutions (they can 'swap' student groups for assessment tasks). However, in many schools this is not possible, so if the relationship is thought to be blurred, the clinical teacher should seek not to assess the particular student involved.

What should clinical teachers assess?

The main strength of assessment in clinical settings is its capacity to assess behaviours and activities in the real world of clinical practice, such as the application of knowledge and skills and the development of professional behaviours. This is where diagnostic reasoning can be 'observed', rather than written about, as case discussions and presentations can show whether or not a student is gathering and processing information appropriately. Similarly, clinical skills can be observed with real patients, ensuring that communication, examination and common procedural skills are developing in the real world. Further, clinical settings are the ideal place to observe ethical and professional behaviour, where students will be observed by many different clinicians and by other health professionals in the healthcare team. Finally, the assessments are closer to the measurement of true *performance*, not just *competence* (*see* Chapter 8), which is consistent with the current trend to find ways of increasing this 'in the real world' assessment and relying less on formal end-point examinations.

The nature of the teacher–student relationship is that clinical teachers may well form views on how well students perform in the whole range of performance aspects. Clinical teachers can contribute to assessments of all of these, although are perhaps better used more strategically.

Scenario 5.3

Each student in the group took turns to present a clinical case verbally during the last two weeks of the clinical rotation, with the order decided at random by the clinical teacher, Dr C. Each student was allocated a patient case, covering several different topics so that the group would learn about several clinical conditions from the series of presentations. On the first designated afternoon, Dr C asked one student to go first, presenting a patient with diabetes. The student was very nervous and stumbled and mumbled through a rather dry presentation. At the end Dr C asked a few questions that the student could not answer. Dr C expressed her frustration, saying: 'If you cannot manage a common case like diabetes, you are going to really struggle in the rest of the course.' Dr C awarded the student 3 out of 10 for the presentation.

While students can be observed in a variety of settings, with many patients and by many different clinical teachers and other health professionals, there are real limitations to this real-world assessment. First, the assessor has to be clear about the focus of the assessment – clinical skills, knowledge of clinical diseases, clinical reasoning, verbal presentation or professional behaviours? All are important and have to be assessed at some stage, but generally not together and perhaps some aspects are better observed by someone other than the main clinical teacher. For example, clinical, communication, procedural and information management skills should be assessed by observation, not by case discussion, and patients and other health professionals can make important contributions to those assessments.

Second, it is difficult to assess clinical knowledge in a series of clinical encounters. Arranging for students to be assessed on the same patients or even the same clinical conditions is very difficult, so students are often assessed on different patients and conditions. This matters less if the focus of the assessment is on clinical skills, rather than knowledge, but does not provide the even playing field that is required of summative assessment. It also highlights the important issue of *context specificity,* meaning that knowledge is often associated with particular patient experiences and patient-based learning. Hence, depending on our learning experiences, we may know a lot about some conditions and less about others. As in Scenario 5.3, it may be possible to know a lot about, say, asthma, because we have encountered quite a lot of patients with it, but we may not have seen many with, say, diabetes, and therefore know much less about that condition. Herein lies one of the major constraints of testing knowledge in clinical settings in just one or two patients; results for students assessed on a relatively narrow range of clinical material can be quite misleading. Even with diabetes – in some ways a 'microcosm of medicine' – it is possible to know well the management of hypertension in non-diabetics and less well its management in diabetics, or vice versa. However, systematic assessment of a broad knowledge base is better achieved through other forms of assessment, such as a well-constructed multiple-choice test.

Third, clinical assessments are logistically complex to conduct with more than one or two patients, due to shortages of patients, observing staff members and time in the real healthcare world. Finally, their role in formative assessment is probably more important at the medical student level, where basic competence is the goal, than in the assessment of experienced professionals, on whom the quality of healthcare rests. These strengths and weaknesses are summarised in Box 5.2.

The common response to these problems is to use assessment in clinical settings to assess certain aspects of performance, such as clinical skills, information management skills and personal and professional behaviours. These are the strengths of real-world assessment and are very difficult in simulated examination settings. Other aspects are assessed in standardised written and clinical examinations that are run centrally. One of the advantages of a well-designed Objective Structured Clinical Examination (OSCE; *see* Chapter 8) is that clinical practice is sampled carefully and widely and student ability is assessed on several different standardised patients with different medical conditions, guided by the curriculum and its learning objectives, thereby providing greater validity and reliability.

Box 5.2 Strengths and weaknesses of student assessment in clinical settings

Strengths
- Ideal for clinical reasoning.
- Ideal for communication skills.
- Ideal for examination skills.
- Ideal for common procedural skills.
- Ideal for ethical, personal and professional behaviours.
- Ideal for information management.
- Ideal for formative assessment.
- Collects views of many clinical teachers.
- Real-world setting.
- Can measure true performance, not just competence.

Weaknesses
- Logistically difficult.
- Limitation to particular setting.

- Case specificity limits extrapolation.
- Less useful in summative assessment.
- Potential problems where assessors disagree.
- Less valuable for broad knowledge base.

Desirable attributes of assessment practices

The terms 'validity' and 'reliability' have so far been used without explanation. They are familiar terms, although often not well understood. Validity is the extent to which an assessment process measures what it intends to measure. Reliability is the extent to which an assessment process, if repeated, would achieve the same result. These are important attributes of assessment, but they are not the only important attributes. There are four others and the six together could be regarded as producing a *utility index* – further details are provided in Chapter 8. Designers of assessment procedures should consider the utility index of the methods and formats before finalising their choice.

Assessment methods commonly used in clinical settings

Clinical teachers are likely to become involved in several forms of assessment of students during clinical placements. Each of these requires a perspective that only those closest to the students can provide.

Short and long clinical cases

These are almost the standard format for assessing clinical skills in most hospital-based disciplines, but have their strengths and weaknesses.

Scenario 5.4

The end of rotation assessment required each student to arrive at 8 am on the Wednesday of the last week, to briefly interview a patient allocated that morning by the registrar at random, and to present the patient to one of the clinical teachers, either Drs D or E, later that day in no more than 30 minutes. The patients came from the wards and included cases of pneumonia, diabetes, early dementia, chronic hepatitis, hypertension, and two with CVAs. Each student presented their patient in the presence of just Dr D or Dr E and an assessment report form was submitted for each patient. The student time involved in each of the cases was approximately one hour.

Scenario 5.5

The end of rotation assessment required each student to arrive at 8 am on the Wednesday of the last week, to interview a patient allocated that

---

Continued

morning by the registrar at random, and to present the patient to one of the clinical teachers, either Drs F or G, later that day in no more than 30 minutes, followed by a detailed discussion of the details of the case. The patients came from the wards and included cases of pneumonia, diabetes, early dementia, chronic hepatitis, hypertension, and two with CVAs. Each student presented their patient in the presence of just Dr F or Dr G and an assessment report form was submitted for each patient. The student time involved in each of the cases was approximately three hours.

These scenarios demonstrate both strengths and weaknesses of clinical cases. They allow for (perhaps prolonged) discussion about clinical topics involving, but not limited to, specific patients. Knowledge and understanding can be explored in depth, including issues not limited by a single case.

On the other hand, they highlight the problem of assessing clinical topics in the absence of direct observation of students performing clinical skills, as in both examples the student conducted the interview and examination alone. This leaves open the possibility that the student might not be proficient at history-taking and examination skills. In many cases this may result in poor performance during the discussion, as in Scenario 5.3, but it may be possible for a confident, verbally skilled student to talk his or her way through a discussion and achieve a passing score without having performed the clinical skills proficiently. Hence it is important to be clear what is being assessed; if clinical skills are to be assessed then students must be observed during clinical encounters.

They also highlight the issue of case specificity. In both scenarios, each student was assessed on different patients, most of whom had different medical problems. This makes it very hard to compare the performance of students with each other, but that is necessary for reliable summative assessment.

On the other hand, reflect on how different Scenarios 5.4 and 5.5 might have been if the purpose of the assessments was purely formative. Each student could receive detailed feedback from the clinical teacher and the other students and, by participating in all cases (mostly as an observer), could learn a lot about several medical conditions in a relatively short time. Hence case presentations are ideal formative assessment methods, and they should be offered several times during clinical education. They can also be used in summative assessment, particularly if they have been used formatively during clinical placements, although logistic feasibility can be a problem where assessing large numbers of students on a reasonable number of patients with different clinical problems. A more current version of the short case assessment is the mini-CEX.

Case studies

A case study is some form of usually written, and sometimes oral, discussion of a particular patient case. Requirements will vary according to the level of the student, but most require the student to interview and examine the patient, read through the patient's files and then synthesise this information into some form of diagnosis and/or management plan, sometimes with integration of basic science or systemic pathology information that explains the patient's problems and management options. Hence a case study can cover a wide range of information and potentially provide information about students' understanding and reasoning. However, it can also be difficult to score and is also relatively easily faked! It also does not allow for assessment of clinical skills, unless they are also observed as part of the assessment process.

Scoring case studies requires understanding of exactly what students are required to do and how to score each part. Both students and clinical teachers should be provided with these details, so that all participants know what is expected. Clinical teachers arguably require more detail on the precise scoring methods, including weightings, etc. for each section, although there is a school of thought that suggests that only global (i.e. overall) scoring be conducted. Global scoring has been shown to be more reliable with experienced teachers and scorers, but may not survive internal appeals processes if a student is unhappy with a score. The most valuable part of the scorer's effort, from the students' perspectives, is the written feedback about what could have been done better. This is the also the most time-consuming and difficult part of the scoring task, but must be done. Clinical teachers involved in scoring case studies should follow the instructions carefully and, if unsure about anything, seek clarification from the medical education unit.

Scenario 5.6

Dr H was asked to score the case studies from another group of eight students. She read the instructions carefully and set to work. By the fifth case study she felt she was seeing things when the case appeared to be very familiar. She looked back and discovered that this case study was about the same patient as in the second case study, and on closer reading found that almost the entire history and examination sections of the two documents were just about identical, including a couple of typographical errors. Much of the other sections were different from each other.

'Faking' has become a complex and controversial topic in written assessment in universities. When is a student's work not his or her own, and how would a scorer know? The generic term 'cheating' appears not to be in favour, but rather the term 'plagiarism'. Plagiarism means that the work is copied from another source without appropriate acknowledgement. This can include citing research findings, copying wording from textbooks or doing a 'cut and paste' from electronic media, including websites, all without appropriate acknowledgement. All of these activities can be acceptable if done infrequently and correctly. Most universities publish guidelines for their students.

When students transgress these guidelines, the only person likely to detect this is the scorer. In Scenario 5.6, the issue is that two students appear to have colluded in writing their case scenarios. Was this because they had to share the same patient because so few were available? What if the collusion was deeper than this? Would the scorer even know if students had inappropriately downloaded and incorporated material from the web? This is much more difficult to detect, although sometimes students will cite 'seminal' works that the scorer recognises. More subtle cases can be identified by special scanning software.

What makes this a particularly difficult issue to sort out is that learners should access, read and cite published works in preparing their case studies! There is a fine line between appropriate and inappropriate citing, and motives can range from none (accidental) and outright cheating (deliberate). Clearly this needs to be explored, and the scorer should refer it to the discipline head or medical education unit rather than taking on personal responsibility.

Increasingly, universities are providing access for both students and teachers to 'anti-plagiarism' software that can measure the degree of match between the written assignments of individual students against those of other students, websites and the academic literature. The match is expressed as a percentage, which may be difficult to interpret, and a decision on just how likely a high match is truly plagiarism still relies on a judgement by the marker. Therefore information from anti-plagiarism software is probably more useful for formative than summative purposes.

Log diaries

Log diaries are widely used to address one of the fundamental problems in clinical teaching. Without guidance, students may not encounter a wide enough range of patients, perform a wide enough range of clinical skills, and therefore learn enough to meet the learning objectives of the course.

Log diaries come in many forms, but usually provide a list of clinical conditions and clinical skills that should be encountered by students. These lists are often divided into two groups – 'core' and 'desirable'. They also might require that students record 'observed', 'supervised' and 'independent' activities, reflecting a gradient in supervision to experience. A common role of clinical teachers is to monitor student progress, as recorded in the log diaries, and to sign off on both individual activities and on satisfactory completion of the process during the clinical rotation.

When used well, log diaries can be very helpful to both students and clinical teachers. They are really a tool to guide learning, particularly the breadth of learning required, and the provision of feedback, based on what has been achieved or not yet achieved.

Log diaries can also be misused, as they are easily manufactured to order. Students can make up entries, copy some from peers, and even obtain forged signatures to individual activities. Such activities are self-delusional, as the main loser is the student who replaces genuine learning with inaccurate or faked entries, and the capacity to succeed depends on how entries are checked. If nobody seems to care what is in a log diary, who can blame students for becoming cynical? Clinical teachers are often in the best place to make log diaries educationally valuable, particularly if they regularly review them with students and use them as a tool in active learning. In this context gaps become learning needs and opportunities, rather than deficiencies.

The use of log diaries in assessment is more controversial. Their main role is in formative assessment, as when used well they can provide useful information about learning progress. On the other hand, their role in summative assessment is less clear. Attempting to use a formative assessment tool in a summative way breaks one of the cardinal rules of assessment: never use information gathered for formative assessment to make decisions about students at barrier examinations.

To do this weakens its role in formative assessment and may even encourage students to manufacture 'evidence' of their progress. Hence if a medical school wants to use log diaries summatively, they really should create one primarily for summative assessment, and then have measures that ensure compliance and minimise cheating. This is not an easy task.

An alternative, and probably more educationally sound, approach is to use a log diary formatively, as described above, and make participation in the process mandatory, without defining a standard for its contents. This still confuses roles a little, but the log diary becomes a 'hurdle' to jump before taking summative assessment, not a contributor to a final score. If done well, this balanced approach can ensure that students actively engage in a valuable learning process.

Learning portfolios

Learning portfolios are part of the new age of teaching and learning in medical education. Many medical schools claim to have such a tool, but closer analysis reveals that this is a very generic term for a wide range of tools that are used in a wide variety of ways. Therefore, before discussing in any detail what a learning portfolio might be used for, three very important questions must be answered.

The first question is: 'what is a learning portfolio?' In simple terms, a learning portfolio is just a collection of learning materials gathered by a learner. This often includes some form of log diary (see above), personal lecture notes, reflections on learning progress and results of formative assessments, etc. A more complete list of possible inclusions is given in Box 5.3. An essential decision for any medical education programme is to define exactly what the learner should include in the learning portfolio for that programme. Inclusions should be relevant to the learning objectives, content and process of the curriculum. Learners should also be free to include materials that they choose to be relevant to their own personal learning. One controversial issue is the relevance of materials on extracurricular activities; while they can contribute a broader view of learners as people, some would argue that personal and professional lives should be kept separate.

Box 5.3 Common inclusions in learning portfolios

- Lists of clinical skills and procedures experienced.
- Personal lecture notes, based on other resources.
- Results of formative assessment.
- Rating forms by self, peers, tutors, patients and health professionals who have contact with the student.
- Copies of identified learning issues with plans for action.
- Evidence-based medicine projects.
- Extra-curricular activities that demonstrate honesty, reliability, ethical behaviour, etc.

The second question is: 'what will the learning portfolio be used for?' This is a crucial question, as the answer will influence the way learners and teachers use learning portfolios. They are most commonly used for formative assessment, as a guide to learners and teachers to the learning progress and mastery of the curriculum. However, if their contents are well matched to the curriculum and learning progress of individual learners, the concept of summative assessment becomes attractive to medical educators. Summative assessment of learning portfolios is a challenging issue that is yet to be clarified in the literature, but increasingly medical schools and postgraduate training programmes are using learning portfolios for summative purposes. The important issue here is that learners must know what will happen to the information they gather and how it will be used to contribute to judgements on their progress.

The third question is: 'why have a learning portfolio?' This is a good question, and one that has not been answered to the satisfaction of some. For medical educators there are two great attractions of requiring students to maintain a learning portfolio. The first is that they can gather information about the progress of students' personal and professional development, as well as clinical performance. Many learning portfolios are evolving into a form of '360 degree' assessment of learners, including how they behave and perform in the real world. Much of that information is difficult to gather and consider in traditional assessment processes. The second attraction is that, as students are responsible for gathering and presenting the information that demonstrates learning progress and achievement, learning portfolios are ideal for encouraging adult learning.

A third issue, really an imperative that supports the use of learning portfolios early in medical education, is that increasingly postgraduate certification and maintenance of registration as a medical practitioner (relicensure or revalidation) requires presentation of a portfolio of evidence that an individual practitioner has maintained knowledge and skills and is of good professional standing. The earlier students start thinking this way, the more prepared they will be for their future roles. Having said that, early medical students often have the most difficulty understanding and using learning portfolios, so simpler, more prescriptive versions and substantial support are needed.

The role of clinical teachers in the learning portfolio process is most likely to be in signing checklists and rating forms on clinical and professional performance of their students. These forms will be included in learning portfolios and may influence decisions about students' progress, so it is an important task that should be conducted with care.

Practical issues in scoring student performance

Much of the written assessment in medical schools is now marked by computer scanning, and the rest is by teams of academics who set the questions and then take time out to score a pile of papers. Clinical teachers may be invited to participate in the latter process, but will most often be asked to contribute by scoring performance of students in case studies and clinical cases that are held either during the rotations or in an OSCE. Attempts are made to objectify and standardise the assessment by asking assessors to complete checklists and rating scales, and to provide detailed written feedback to be passed on to students. A further request is often made for comments on the assessment items or the assessment process itself; this is to assist the medical education unit on quality control assessment processes.

Checklists

A checklist is a list of what should happen and records whether or not each one did happen. This usually results in a yes (a mark is awarded) or no (zero marks) result for each line. The total score for the station is derived by adding up the 'yes' box scores. Students can then receive both a total score and feedback about what they did or did not do. Checklists are simple, but their weakness is that they are better at measuring that things happen than how well they are done. Some assessors find this dissatisfying, as an 'all or nothing' approach may not suit all the scoring of aspects of performance. To partly overcome this, a middle column is sometimes added so that part marks can be awarded for doing the expected activity, but not well enough to deserve full marks. This still requires a judgement by the assessor, something that inexperienced assessors find difficult. The more that the checklist categories describe exactly what the student is expected to do for each mark, the easier the task becomes. Sometimes generic checklists are used for clinical stations, leaving some lines as 'not applicable' in certain cases, and not necessarily precisely defining what is expected for the marks. Ideally, each checklist is designed specifically for its station, and therefore every line is relevant, clearly described and scored. An example of a simple checklist specifically designed for assessment of how to record an electrocardiogram (ECG) is provided in Figure 5.1.

Marking guide for station cardiac clinical station	Performed competently	Performed but not fully competent	Not performed or incompetent
Washed hands	2	1	0
Correct placing of ECG electrodes	4	2	0
Adequate recording	2	1	0
Clear explanation to patient	3	1.5	0
Explains ECG is normal	3	2	0
Suggests follow-up	1	0.5	0

Total / 15

Figure 5.1 An example of a checklist for performing an ECG on a patient.

Rating scales

Rating scales allow assessors to judge how well a candidate performs at the stated task. For each desired attribute or behaviour, there is a sliding scale with points that indicate degrees of quality of performance. There are two kinds of scales. The first uses numbers to indicate the intervals, from 1 (absent) to a number indicating perfect, usually from 5 to 10. This is called a Likert scale. Sometimes the polarity of the scales is reversed, such that 1 means excellent and 10 means absent – it is wise to read the instructions carefully. The second kind uses verbal descriptors to define intervals; terms such as 'extremely poor', 'poor', 'acceptable', 'very good' and 'excellent' are commonly used. These are called semantic differential scales or behaviourally anchored rating scales (BARS). The descriptors should describe, as well as is feasible, the actual behaviour which merits that rating. The better the description of the behaviour at each point, the easier they are to use and the more reliable the result. The use of 'very poor' to 'excellent' is less meaningful. Behavioural anchors are also sometimes used in conjunction with Likert scales. Examples of both are provided in Figure 5.2.

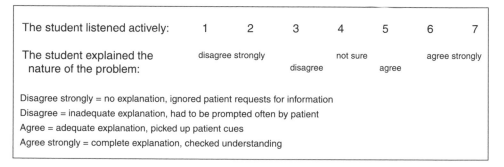

Figure 5.2 Examples of numerical and semantic differential rating scales.

Rating scales also have inbuilt problems that pose challenges, particularly for inexperienced assessors. The best way to use rating scales is to consider each line separately and make a judgement about how well the student performed in that particular aspect or behaviour. Some students will quite frankly deserve the lowest possible rating for some aspects or behaviours. At the other end of the scale, some will do everything just perfectly and deserve the highest rating. The majority will be somewhere in between most of the time.

There are several interesting patterns in scoring rating scales that should be avoided. The first is where an assessor starts with the assumption that the mid-point is where most students probably lie and they tend to score at the mid-point most frequently. For better performance the assessor moves up a point, for worse performance down a point, but the extremes are rarely used. A variation of this is where an assessor knows that the 'pass' score is really at, say, point 5 of a 7-point scale, and tends to cluster scores around that point. This is known as 'central tendency marking' and results in student scores being very close to each other, all around the middle or 'pass' score.

The second is where an assessor scores everybody poorly and then complains about falling standards. Scores for individual aspects or behaviours will be at the bottom of the scale, with perhaps an occasional score around the middle. This kind of assessor is known as a 'hawk'. The third is the opposite to a 'hawk' – a 'dove'. This kind of assessor believes that all students should pass and tends to score every student in the upper end of the scale. The problem with both 'hawks' and 'doves' is one of calibration; neither is attuned to the expected standards of the group of learners, with either too high or too low expectations. To some extent, this may also be a personality issue; 'hawks' are often very judgemental. Both 'hawks' and 'doves' can still be examiners, as with feedback they might change. If they persist with their approach, they can be paired with an assessor of the opposite persuasion, so that through discussion final results

> **(1 = agree strongly; 2 = agree; 3 = agree a little; 4 = unsure; 5 = disagree a little; 6 = disagree; 7 = disagree strongly)**

a. Central tendency scoring

The student:

was punctual	1	2	3	④	5	6	7
attended scheduled teaching sessions	1	2	3	4	5	6	7
dressed appropriately for clinical work	1	2	3	4	5	6	7
demonstrated respect for patients' needs	1	2	3	4	5	6	7
made legible contributions to patients' files	1	2	3	4	5	6	7
recognised own limits	1	2	3	4	5	6	7

b. 'Hawkish' marking

The student:

was punctual	1	2	3	4	5	6	⑦
attended scheduled teaching sessions	1	2	3	4	5	⑥	7
dressed appropriately for clinical work	1	2	3	4	5	⑥	⑦
demonstrated respect for patients' needs	1	2	3	4	5	6	7
made legible contributions to patients' files	1	2	3	4	5	6	7
recognised own limits	1	2	3	4	5	⑥	7

c. 'Dovish' marking

The student:

was punctual	①	2	3	4	5	6	7
attended scheduled teaching sessions	①	2	3	4	5	6	7
dressed appropriately for clinical work	1	②	3	4	5	6	7
demonstrated respect for patients' needs	1	②	3	4	5	6	7
made legible contributions to patients' files	①	2	3	4	5	6	7
recognised own limits	①	2	3	4	5	6	7

d. Halo marking

The student:

was punctual	1	2	3	4	5	6	7
attended scheduled teaching sessions	1	2	3	4	5	6	7
dressed appropriately for clinical work	1	2	3	4	5	6	7
demonstrated respect for patients' needs	1	2	3	4	5	6	7
made legible contributions to patients' files	1	2	3	4	5	6	7
recognised own limits	1	2	3	4	5	6	7

e. Appropriate scoring

The student:

was punctual	1	②	3	4	5	6	7
attended scheduled teaching sessions	1	2	③	4	5	6	7
dressed appropriately for clinical work	1	2	3	4	5	⑥	7
demonstrated respect for patients' needs	1	2	3	4	5	6	⑦
made legible contributions to patients' files	①	2	3	4	5	6	7
recognised own limits	1	2	3	4	5	⑥	7

Figure 5.3 Examples of common patterns in scoring rating scales.

end up as a compromise. However, some 'hawks' and 'doves' cannot work together like that.

A fourth pattern is 'halo marking' where an assessor allows a judgement of one aspect of performance to affect judgement of other aspects. For example, if the student is 'nice' to a simulated or real patient, and therefore scored at the highest level for interpersonal skills, an assessor might not notice that important aspects of history taking are omitted or done poorly, and score the particular student highly on all aspects. The opposite can also occur, with low scores being given for all aspects or behaviours because one or two are done poorly.

The ideal pattern is no pattern; that is, all points in the scale, including the extremes, are used on occasion for most students. Examples of these patterns are provided in Figure 5.3. Correct standard setting and calibration of assessors (through training and experience) produces better scoring.

There are two further problems encountered in scoring rating scales. The first is that they are tiring to complete several times in a row over a short period of time, and attention can waver. It is possible for several students to become a blurred group, with an assessor not sure what the current student has or has not done. This is best addressed by taking regular breaks from scoring. OSCEs frequently have 'rest' stations; most people think they are for the students, but rests for assessors are equally important. Examinations should be organised so that assessors do not get fatigued.

The final issue is called 'black-balling'. This is where an assessor decides that poor performance in one aspect equals an automatic overall fail, regardless of how well other aspects are performed. For example, should a student completely miss a diagnosis, or perhaps fail to intubate a model patient safely, or recommend a dangerous dose of a drug, then the consequences in real life of such lapses cause some examiners to believe firmly that the student should fail, regardless of performance elsewhere in the assessments. This is always a contentious issue, but the correct approach is not to fail a student on the basis of a single 'important' lack of knowledge or skill. Important skills such as cardiopulmonary resuscitation (CPR) skills can instead be made 'hurdles' to be completed satisfactorily (and can be repeated until they are) prior to commencing other scored assessments.

Providing detailed feedback

Arguably the most educationally important part of any assessment is the description of what the student did or did not do. This is particularly helpful when performance is not as strong as it should be, as it guides learning and improvement. Without this feedback, students will often complain that they do not know how they could have done any better.

Hence it is essential that assessors write down as much detail as possible about the performance. Include what actually happened (if it was not correct) and, where possible, advice on how to improve. If there is no room on the front of the scoring sheet (there should be room for examiner comments), turn over and write it on the back. This is the most time-consuming part of the assessment role and it sometimes has to fit into just one to two minutes between students. If not done at the time, the students will become a blur and specific comments will be difficult to recall and ascribe to particular students.

Quality control

The achievement of a high-quality assessment process, both individual assessment items and the overall process, is a very important goal for medical schools. It is important that students are treated fairly and correct decisions are made. The medical education unit will want to hear about any concerns assessors might have about scoring problems, possible semantic confusion or ambiguous or redundant wording in items, or any other difficulties. Often space will be provided for these comments but, if not, either write them down or send them in later.

Pass/fail mechanisms in student assessment

The key decision in any assessment process is whether or not a student has achieved a high enough score to allow progress to the next year of the course and, ultimately, to obtain a university degree. Determining this passing or 'cut-off' score is at the heart of assessment processes. This is discussed in more detail in Chapter 8, where standard-setting procedures are briefly explained.

Despite the importance of the pass/fail decision, traditional reporting of assessment scores is often more concerned with ranking students from top to bottom and categorising their performance as distinctions or credits, etc. Medical students are often high achievers who thrive on such feedback and the choice of postgraduate careers can depend on the level of academic performance.

However, many of the newer curricula have changed from grading and ranking scores to an apparently simpler, non-graded, 'pass/fail' system. This has sound educational reasoning at its core, in that it fosters collaborative learning and focuses on the most important cutting score – pass or fail. Potential advantages are that students become used to being part of a team, as they will have to be in the future, and will assist each other, rather than strive for individual excellence at the expense of peers. Tales abound of textbooks and other resources disappearing around examination time to give the 'borrower' an advantage over the rest. However, like most education initiatives, it can have some unwanted consequences. These include concerns that it also fosters complacency in some students, who rarely fear failure, but will cease to strive for excellence. Non-graded assessment also does not satisfy students who are driven by success and being at the top of the cohort, academically speaking.

Where non-graded assessment is instituted, it must be accompanied by strong formative assessment processes that clearly indicate to students how they are performing in relation to criterion-referenced standards. As a compromise between the two models, detailed private feedback can also be provided to students on their performance, including actual scores and perhaps the quartile in which their scores lie. This still allows students to work collaboratively, without public rankings of performance, but ensures that students at both the borderline and the top know in more detail just how they are performing.

The implications for clinical teachers are that they should understand and accept the decisions of medical schools about their pass/fail judgement mechanisms, and they should focus on making the most accurate judgements they can, and then provide the most detailed, specific feedback to help students understand their strengths and weaknesses. Whatever the assessment process, these are important roles for clinical teachers.

Making and living with the best judgement

Assessors are human and can only do their best when making a judgement about a student's abilities. The more experienced the assessor, the better they know what is expected of students at all levels, and the more valid and reliable will be their judgements.

A common dilemma faced by assessors, particularly those who get to know students well, is what to do if the performance of a student appears to be poor. It may be that their prior knowledge of the student causes the assessor to believe that the student 'deserves better'. Others might find the performance too close to the borderline to award a low (failing) score. Quite often students are given the benefit of the doubt and end up with a borderline, although just good enough score that allows them to proceed. Assessors sometimes salve their consciences by assuming that these students will either improve or be picked up by the next assessor – after all, surely students should not be held up because of the judgement of just one assessor?

Sadly, this is how students with problems manage to get quite a long way into a course before persistent problems are discovered and dealt with. Such problems can be with professional behaviour, knowledge or skills. For assessment in clinical settings, the emphasis should be on professional behaviours and clinical skills, and clinical teachers have a particular responsibility to ensure that they identify, try to fix and report any weakness in students. The sooner these problems are dealt with, the easier they are to remedy. Medical schools have a real dilemma on their hands when serious deficiencies are found in senior students.

Hence the simple advice to clinical teachers is to make judgements to the best of their ability. If the judgement is that a student is not performing well, then so be it. Clinical teachers may feel disappointed, but should never feel guilty for making and reporting such a judgement. The medical school should have processes that will deal with these situations.

Summary

This chapter has briefly addressed several issues that explain the importance of assessment in clinical teaching, and provides examples of assessment practices to guide clinical teachers to develop their assessment skills.

Further reading

- Dornan T, Carroll C and Parboosingh J (2002) An electronic learning portfolio for reflective continuing professional development. *Medical Education.* **36**: 767–9.
  Reports the challenges of using electronic learning portfolios, despite the eagerness of some.
- Webb C, Endacott R, Gray M *et al.* (2002) Models of portfolios. *Medical Education.* **36**: 897–8.
  Light-hearted look at learning portfolio formats.

Chapter 6

Evaluating clinical teaching and learning

> There is a measure in things.
> Horace, *c*.65–68 BC

Introduction

Just as sound clinicians are interested in the quality of their medical care, and participate in attempts to measure their clinical practice, so too should clinical teachers be interested in the quality of their teaching. It is difficult to stop learners learning, but more difficult to ensure that learners are proceeding down the right learning pathways. As with the measurement of the quality of healthcare, the measurement of teaching quality can be a very complex, multi-perspective task that may include many different approaches.

Medical schools generally conduct two kinds of teaching quality assessment. The first is the less complex, more reflexive measurement of student opinion. This form of assessment, often just called student feedback, is an important part of curriculum implementation, because it provides academic staff with some idea of how well received their courses are, at least in the eyes of their consumers, the students. Collecting student feedback also sends messages to students that their views are welcome, so long as students can see changes resulting from their feedback. The second kind of quality assessment is more formal programme evaluation, which measures how well the course is meeting educational objectives, internal university practices and external (national and sometimes international) benchmarks.

Programme evaluation is a substantial topic that is probably of less interest to clinical teachers. They are more interested in measuring how well they teach their own students, so this chapter focuses on the practical issues relevant to that task.

Why measure teaching quality?

The obvious answer to such a question is that novice teachers need to know how to develop expertise and sound teachers want and deserve affirmation of their expertise. Educational institutions generally adopt a continuous quality improvement (CQI) model, whereby teaching staff members regularly consider their teaching performance and strive to improve, whatever their level of performance.

Hence the main purpose of teaching evaluations is formative, or to provide feedback to teachers and the medical school as a promoter of improvement. Teaching evaluations can also be summative, in that academic staff members may seek evidence to support promotion or, infrequently, evidence to avoid disciplinary action for alleged poor performance. Please note the similarity of the language with that of student assessment, but here the teacher, not the students, is the subject of the measurement. Chapter 8 provides more detail on the theoretical approach to measurements.

Please note also the use of the term 'evaluation', rather than 'assessment'. By definition, evaluation is measurement against a standard, for a purpose. This concept is important for two reasons. First, it indicates that teacher performance can be compared not just with other measures of the same teacher, but against the performance of other teachers. Standards are less well defined for teaching quality than for student performance, but most clinical teachers would accept that it is possible to define poor teaching practices and to strive to eliminate them. The second importance is that the purpose of teacher evaluations, as with student assessment, should always be clear, and that formative evaluations should not be used summatively.

If teacher performance is measured against a standard, then recognition is possible for those teachers judged to have met or exceeded the desired standard. Such recognition, with rewards, is highly desirable to encourage quality improvement.

Measures of teaching quality

> **Scenario 6.1**
>
> Dr A, a clinical teacher with 10 years' experience, reflected on his experience with the just completed third clinical rotation for the year. This was the first year of a new curriculum that he had helped to create by attendance at curriculum planning meetings. The first two groups seemed to go well – there was a lot of discussion about the new curriculum and how different the students might be, but they seemed to have a positive experience and to reach the expected standard. However, the last group had a lot of trouble and he had actually failed two of the six students in their case presentations. He was genuinely puzzled over how this happened. He wanted to know what he could have done better.

In Scenario 6.1 it is not easy to determine where the problem may lie. However, Dr A could, if he wanted, seek more information and try to find out.

One of the dilemmas in measuring the quality of teaching is that there are many variables in the equation, many co-dependent, and some not able to be influenced by the clinical teacher.

Let us begin with the variables that the clinical teacher cannot influence, or influence to any substantial degree. The first is the curriculum, which is imposed by the medical school. No matter how consultative the medical curriculum planners were, there is no such thing as a perfect curriculum that is 100% supported by 100% of the core academic and clinical teaching staff. By necessity, curricula have to achieve a lot with limited time and resources, so inevitably there is debate about what is included or excluded.

The second is the choice of students in the group allocated to the clinical teacher. As a group, medical students may be academically bright and motivated, but they come with different personalities, different life experiences and variable levels of interest in particular disciplines. They also come at different times of the academic year, and most experienced clinical teachers recognise that students who have done other clinical rotations are usually more proficient than those at the beginning of their first clinical rotation.

The third is the clinical workload available for learning during any particular clinical rotation. Clinical units tend to be busy all of the time, and over a year the case-mix may be similar, but within any shorter period, usually several weeks, patients may not necessarily reflect the focus of the curriculum.

Therefore there are some issues that, while important to the measurement of the quality of the overall teaching programme, are much less relevant to the quality of the contribution of individual clinical teachers. However, there are several variables to which clinical teachers can make a contribution and their measurement can potentially offer information about their teaching expertise. These are listed in Box 6.1.

Attendance and punctuality of students could be proxy measures for the degree to which a teacher interests the students and motivates them to attend. However, as discussed in earlier chapters, these behaviours can also be evidence of student problems, such as poor physical and mental health, or other personal problems. Similarly, lack of participation of individual students in teaching sessions can reflect poor small group process skills on the part of the teacher, but can also be due to a few students having more introverted personalities.

Box 6.1 Measures of teaching quality

- Attendance and punctuality of students.
- Participation in teaching activities of students.
- Student evaluations.
- Peer evaluations.
- Expert evaluations.
- Self-assessment results.
- Assessment results.
- Future student progress.

The more direct measures of individual teacher performance come from the students and from those who observe student–teacher interactions. Students' assessments usually focus on satisfaction, which is a curious and complex construct of issues that are certainly important, but difficult to tease apart. Rating forms can attempt this by having separate scales for attendance, punctuality, respect, communication skills, etc., but students often rate their clinical teachers globally, with the halo phenomenon evident where they like the clinical teacher (*see* Chapter 5 for more on interpreting rating scales).

Peer evaluations can be very valuable, as they are judgements made by people doing the same job and therefore aware of the challenges and constraints. Ideally, they are based on observation of one or several teaching sessions and involve the completion of a rating scale that provides the basis of feedback. Many clinical teachers will welcome and act on the advice of their peers. A sound model is for a whole group of clinical teachers to arrange to observe each other's teaching sessions. One way of doing this is for a pair of clinical teachers to observe each other, and then discuss what they learned. Another way is for clinical teachers to observe another, but to be observed by a different person, and then the whole group discuss what they learned. As with all external judgement and accreditation processes, the observer probably learns more about his or her own teaching than the person being observed, so the critical requirement is that all clinical teachers observe another.

Evaluations by 'experts' means that course coordinators, or some other external person, may observe a clinical teacher, complete a rating scale of some kind and make judgements about a teacher's performance compared with their deeper knowledge of the role and perhaps wider experience with teaching in other, similar settings.

Self-assessment by clinical teachers can be valuable, but also quite challenging. As with performance in clinical practice, awareness of one's own strengths and weaknesses as a teacher is an essential part of developing true expertise. Self-awareness develops from assimilation of feedback from others (students, peers and experts), but can be facilitated by observation of one's own performance as a teacher. The best way of observing one's own performance is to audiotape or videotape a teaching session. The students must give their consent and all must accept that any analysis of the recording will not have any impact on student assessments. The power of self-observation is that we see ourselves from another perspective. It is common to be worried about appearance, voice and mannerisms, and to be a harsher critic than other observers, but once that has been accepted, we can learn from comparing our own performance with our understanding of the role and how others perform.

The results of student assessments are a crude measure of teacher performance, but only if there are consistent results over several groups. It is possible for poor teaching to be a cause of poor student performance, but this is an unlikely outcome, partly because students usually recognise when they may be disadvantaged, report it to the medical school, and seek ways of making up for perceived disadvantages through working with other students in their own time. However, using student assessment results is at least an attempt to measure the impact on learning of the teaching.

Scenario 6.2

At the graduation dinner several just-completing students were reminiscing about their experiences in the clinical years and what they might want to do after internship. One volunteered that one of her most vivid memories was Dr B, a depressed GP tutor who often told her that the practice of any medical discipline was not the job it used to be and that, in particular, general practice was a 'dead end'. Others laughed and related similar experiences with Dr B. They agreed that it was sad that Dr B was so depressed, but all felt that they would not consider a general practice career as a result of his consistent negativity.

The final potential measure that may be discussed is the future progress of students. Many clinical teachers feel quite proud when their former students go on to do great things and may even feel a degree of credit for these outcomes. The link is tenuous at best, although very good teachers and role models can inspire students to do well in the future, often within their own discipline or specialty. The reverse may also be true; that is, very poor role models may demotivate students, as in Scenario 6.2. If most students exposed to a particular clinical teacher are totally uninspired, the clinical teacher probably needs a vacation, antidepressants or retirement! Unfortunately, this is a very long-term indicator; course coordinators should detect and deal with such situations before too much harm is done.

A practical approach to evaluating your teaching

Should clinical teachers wish to obtain a formal evaluation of their clinical teaching, there are two broad approaches: using existing student evaluation processes and developing a more individual evaluation process.

Existing student evaluation processes

Most universities have centres for teaching and learning, or organisations with similar titles. These centres provide advice to all faculties and schools on teaching and learning issues and usually conduct campus-wide student feedback surveys. They also have teaching feedback processes that individual academic staff may use. These processes usually include surveys of teachers by student groups, but they are also usually designed for the more traditional university model of stable teaching staff teaching on campus over a whole semester or even a year. Medical courses, particularly in more senior years, tend to place students in contact with a large number of clinical teachers at several sites, so course teaching evaluations are very blunt instruments for working out how well individual teachers perform. Most medical schools have medical education units and the staff in those units are likely to have evaluation processes more oriented to clinical teaching, including rating forms more suitable for part-time teachers, so long as the contact hours between the teacher and the students allow for students to make reasonable judgements.

Developing individual evaluation processes

Where the university or medical school does not have evaluation processes relevant to clinical teaching, individual clinical teachers can, with a little help, design or adapt evaluation processes that provide useful information. These are summarised in Box 6.2, and should be seen as a somewhat idealistic approach that would be too complex to implement in total, but should be regarded as a 'toolbox' of potentially useful evaluation processes.

A questionnaire to all students sounds like a reasonable idea, but questionnaire design is quite an art that requires very close attention to semantics of the questions. Further, the number of students to respond is likely to be small, so a quantitative approach is difficult. Instead, the most valuable information may come from asking open-ended questions or seeking three most positive and least positive aspects of the teacher's performance, although this requires qualitative analysis skills for analysis. Focus groups of students are a much less structured way of gathering more open-ended information about what the students thought and felt, but they need to be managed by a person experienced in focus group methods. The clinical teacher should not be involved in the groups, an experienced facilitator is needed and both questionnaires and focus group tapes need transcription and analysis by a qualitative methodologist, so substantial resources are required. Therefore while these methods are possible, clinical teachers should get some advice before going too far. On the other hand, a more pragmatic approach might provide useful information with fewer resources, so long as information is not over-interpreted.

Box 6.2 A toolbox of processes for evaluating clinical teaching

- Questionnaire survey.
- Focus groups.
- Ask a peer to observe your teaching.
- Offer to observe a peer teaching.
- Recording a teaching session.

As discussed above, arranging for clinical teachers to observe each other is a very useful teaching development process and can also provide information on the quality of an individual teacher's performance, along with guidance on how to improve. Finally, recording a teaching session, with consent of all participants, can improve self-awareness of teaching performance, particularly if a peer or a respected 'expert' clinical teacher also observes the recording and discusses any issues with the recorded clinical teacher.

Returning to Scenario 6.1, Dr A then should seek advice from the medical education unit of the medical school in order to answer his question. For a start, they may know more about this group of students, as it is possible that they have developed, or will develop, a reputation for being a 'difficult group'. There are likely to be 'off the shelf' teaching evaluation processes that the unit could recommend, as well as advice on how to adapt processes or develop more specific processes to answer Dr A's question.

Self-observing of teaching sessions

A simple, yet brave, method of reflecting on one's teaching practices is to record and then observe a teaching encounter. Video recording is potentially more powerful, as it captures the non-verbal behaviours so well, but can be more intrusive. Audio recording is simpler and less intrusive, and can still provide a lot of information.

There are some simple 'rules' to follow in this activity. Students (and patients, if they are involved) must give formal consent, ideally in writing. Try to be yourself, and remember that after a few minutes most participants forget that they are being recorded, so the fear of artificiality is somewhat overstated. Choose a quiet time to observe/listen to the recording. Rate your performance using some form of rating scale (an example of a simple formative rating scale is given in Figure

6.1, although not all issues are relevant to all teaching sessions). Ideally, ask someone else to also observe and comment (possibly using the same rating scale) on your performance; this could be a colleague (perhaps you could both do this and comment on each other's recordings?). A respected senior colleague or a member of the medical education unit might also offer interesting perspectives. If you are really brave, also ask one of the students to do this. Think about any differences between comments and ratings between others and yourself. Ask yourself questions such as: Are there any patterns? What did I do well? What did not seem to work? What could I do better next time?

A less threatening method is to ask a colleague to sit in and observe your teaching session and then give feedback later. This is also an activity for pairs of clinical teachers to do with each other's teaching sessions, but it lacks the power of self-evaluation.

	Disagree				Agree
The learning objectives of the session were clear	1	2	3	4	5
Students appeared to be relaxed and involved	1	2	3	4	5
Students all participated actively	1	2	3	4	5
Students were encouraged to ask questions	1	2	3	4	5
Students were guided rather than dominated	1	2	3	4	5
Students were frequently asked questions	1	2	3	4	5
Answers to questions probed learning further	1	2	3	4	5
Audiovisual presentations were clear	1	2	3	4	5
Roles of other health professionals were discussed	1	2	3	4	5
Ethical and legal issues were discussed	1	2	3	4	5
Key learning points were summarised clearly	1	2	3	4	5
'Homework' was identified and allocated	1	2	3	4	5
Follow-up was arranged to deal with questions	1	2	3	4	5
Overall performance:	1	2	3	4	5
The three most positive features were:					
The three least positive features were:					

Figure 6.1 A simple teaching session assessment tool.

Common pitfalls in teaching evaluation

Most teaching evaluations will of necessity be relatively simple processes that provide raw or semi-processed information to clinical teachers for absorption and reflection. Evaluation methodologists would point out that any such information needs careful consideration and interpretation, linked back to the original questions and the methods used. A useful analogy may be to consider the differences between a high-stakes externally funded clinical research project and an in-house pilot project that cannot access expert methodologists. The latter provides useful information, but not the 'final' answer.

This section therefore presents some issues that clinical teachers should be aware of in interpreting their teaching evaluations.

Placing too much emphasis on a particular student group

As indicated previously, student group membership can be a 'wild card' variable. If students are allocated centrally in a random manner, then group dynamics will depend on how complete or relative strangers work out how to cooperate, allocate tasks and share contributions to group activities. They will need guidance in small group processes, and most groups will work out well. Things may not work out so well if a particular group 'accidentally' includes two or three dominant individuals who compete for control, or too many introverts who try to merge with the décor and say very little.

If students organise their own groups, a common situation with more senior medical students, then some groups will be a collection of close friends who work well together, although may also work too well together, in that they share the work too much and do less as individuals than desired. A worse situation arises when the group comprises the 'leftovers' – students who do not get on well with any others and who tend to function as individualists. Such groups show little cohesion and may include students with personal and/or professional behaviour concerns. This is often a group that attracts concern from several different teachers, both full-time medical school staff and clinical teachers in hospitals and practices.

Having acknowledged that student groups are variable in the way they form and function, blaming a particular group of students for problems that arise can be too easy a way out. Rather than shrugging the shoulders and looking forward to the next group, clinical teachers should try to learn from the experience of dealing with a difficult group. As discussed in Chapter 4, small group process skills are essential and indeed able to be developed. Even if a clinical teacher has a 'bad' group, improving group process skills can result in improved group function.

Placing insufficient emphasis on a particular student group

While it is most unlikely that an entire year cohort of students would be much different from other cohorts, within-year group variations are more likely. It is possible for 'the group from hell' to somehow form and continue in a dysfunctional manner. Course organisers should consider this possibility if a group receives consistent criticism from several different clinical teachers. There are two concerns in such a situation. The first is that some clinical teachers can lose the motivation to teach if they do not enjoy the task, and it is possible for a particularly unrewarding experience with a dysfunctional group to result in withdrawal from teaching. The second concern is for the learning of the group. It is most unlikely that all members of a dysfunctional group are poor students, but is quite likely that most will learn less that they should within their group. Clinical teachers should report concerns about a particular group to the course organiser. Should this be yet another report from a sound clinical teacher about a group that is developing a reputation, then the course organiser should step in and investigate the group function. Sometimes allocation of an experienced clinical teacher will improve the group dynamics and the learning environment, but occasionally group membership might have to be changed.

Individual students are at fault

This issue is a corollary to the poor group situation. As a rule, by the time they get to senior course years, individual students are usually not the cause of serious problems. The most likely cause of a single occurrence of a poor relationship between a student and a clinical teacher is a personality conflict. If the same student has several clashes with different clinical teachers, he or she may well have a personal problem that needs to be sorted out. Similarly, if the same clinical teacher has several clashes with different students, he or she may need to be called aside for some discussion about motivation and teaching style. Neither situation is common, and both are likely to be due to loss of motivation, or an emerging physical or mental health problem.

The curriculum is at fault

As a general rule, if a whole year cohort of students performs unexpectedly poorly, compared to previous groups in the same course, then the most likely cause is poor implementation of the curriculum or assessment procedures, not that 'this year's students are not as good as the last few'.

Having acknowledged that 'truism', the issue is just what part of a curriculum process might be at fault. Curricula receive a lot of criticism, largely because there are almost always compromises between the demands of many groups. There is no such thing as the ideal medical curriculum (*see* Chapter 7).

A curriculum document is really a kind of road map, defining the beginning, the route and the end of a learning journey. However, the journey depends on many things other than the curriculum document, such as how the curriculum is implemented and assessed. Implementation can be affected by several factors, such as the quality of the clinical teaching, including the range of clinical material encountered, the number of patients interviewed and examined, the coaching and supervision of clinical skills, the quality of feedback given and role modelling (indeed, all those issues covered in Chapters 3 and 4). The match of assessment to curriculum is also important.

Hence there is plenty of scope for individuals to feel that the curriculum is the problem, but the real issue is to identify which part of the curriculum and assessment processes might be a concern. Most often any problems lie with the how, rather than the what.

On the other hand, consistent concerns about the same aspects of a curriculum are a useful source of information for course organisers. Common threads often indicate a genuine problem, so they should be explored and, if proven, amended.

It won't make any difference anyway

Clinical teachers may feel so distant from the coordination of clinical teaching that they feel as if their comments will not make a difference. This is more likely to happen if the staffing structure does not encourage clinical teachers to feel, and be, part of the academic team. If clinical teachers feel disempowered, they may not pass on the kind of information referred to above that might indicate that a group, an individual student or a curriculum component is possibly a problem. Clinical teachers should pass this information on as medical education units will take it seriously and investigate the need for change.

Summary

This chapter has provided a very brief introduction to teaching evaluations. All clinical teachers should participate in these processes, primarily for the purpose of improving their teaching expertise, based on the feedback received from students, peers and expert observers. The next two chapters, in Part 3 of the book, provide a more detailed and theoretical approach of common issues in teaching and learning, and the methodology of assessment and evaluation.

Further reading

- Best JW and Kahn JV (1989) *Research in Education* (5e). Prentice-Hall, Englewood Cliffs, NJ.
  An overview of approaches to educational research and evaluation. Full of practical examples from classroom settings.
- Donabedian A (1988) The quality of care: how can it be assessed? *Journal of the American Medical Association.* **260**: 1743–8.
  A clear explanation of the most often cited model of evaluation in healthcare.

Part 3

Understanding clinical teaching

Chapter 7

What can be learnt in clinical settings?

> The art of medicine consists of amusing the patient while Nature cures the disease.
>
> Voltaire (attributed), 1694–1778

Introduction

Curricula come in many different forms and use a lot of educational jargon and complex conceptual diagrams. This chapter places clinical teaching within the context of a medical school curriculum, presents some key theoretical concepts relevant to curriculum development and implementation, and provides explanations of commonly used educational terms. This material may be useful in gaining a deeper understanding of why and how various educational strategies might succeed or fail, and can be read either before or after the practical approach taken in Part 2. Depending on personality style and learning style preference, some clinical teachers may wish to achieve a better understanding of the origins of the tasks they are given by the medical school.

Curriculum structure

Overview

To begin with, consider the whole curriculum process. This is much simpler than many think. There should be a list of what needs to be learned (what many think is the curriculum), how this might be done (implementation), and how students are shown to have learned the list to a satisfactory degree (assessment). Ideally, it also includes how to determine if the curriculum is achieving what it intended (evaluation).

What makes a curriculum complex is the detail. Curriculum content is potentially huge, as there is a lot of knowledge and skills needed for competent medical practice. However, the amount of content necessary for a medical student course is a lot less than the total available for inclusion and the necessary elements for this level of learning need to be selected, ideally guided by the goals and objectives of the medical course. The selected content must be organised into *domains* or *themes* (*see* p. 111). Learning objectives are then developed to guide the implementation and assessment. Implementation (or delivery) is then planned for this selected and organised curriculum content. The choice of implementation methods is guided by the content and the learning objectives. The impact on the students of the selected curriculum content by the chosen delivery methods is assessed by measurement of how well they have achieved the learning objectives, which are also the assessment objectives. This overall structure is summarised in Figure 7.1.

The rest of this chapter focuses on the choice and organisation of curriculum content. Assessment and evaluation issues are essential components of a curriculum, and are dealt with in more detail in Chapter 8.

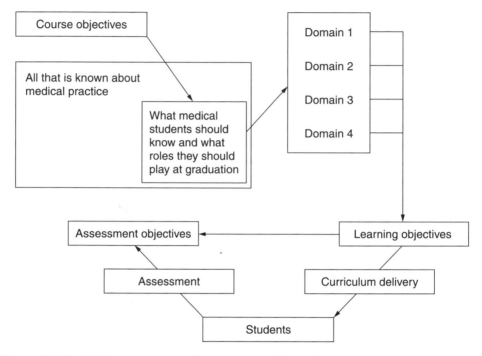

Figure 7.1 Curriculum structure and component relationships.

Defining curriculum content

Deciding on just what is included in a curriculum for medical students is a remarkably complex task. There is so much that could be there, particularly if curriculum planners do not keep in sight the goals of the medical programme. These goals are usually agreed for an entire jurisdiction by the relevant national or, increasingly, regional jurisdiction. For Australia and New Zealand, this organisation is the Australian Medical Council. In North America, Canada and the USA also work together, as do most nations in the European Union (EU), although the recent expansion of the EU has posed challenges as Europe now includes so many different medical education and healthcare systems. The United Kingdom (UK) has a combination of individual and European regulations, but has its own governing body, the General Medical Council.

Most of these jurisdictions define standards of exit from medical education programmes; these standards generally reflect a range of stakeholder views – funders, employers and broader community groups – in addition to those of the medical profession. For medical schools, the standard required is competence to commence, under supervision and in an accredited teaching hospital, early postgraduate training in a chosen specialty. Hence medical school curricula are required to provide only a basic platform on which to build postgraduate and continuing professional development levels.

Medical school curricula are always criticised for not having enough content for most postgraduate careers, and of course that is correct. Typically, the content of a curriculum is fiercely debated right down to the last detail, dealing with conflicting views from several professional organisations that may have strong views on the amount of detail required. For example, should graduates from medical school know the principles of cancer treatment, or should they know the cytotoxic regimes for the commonest forms of cancer? Most medical schools would argue against the latter, as this kind of detail is readily available and is likely to change before the new graduates are in positions of responsibility where they might prescribe management plans. If all advice were followed, an under-graduate curriculum would be 20 years long and would include enough information for registration in several specialties. In this stage of curriculum design, the hardest question is what to leave out. Clinicians participating in a major curriculum development will have a lot of fun witnessing some interesting turf wars.

Organising curriculum content

There are several ways of organising the selected curriculum content. Simple methods include lists of desired topics, in varying degrees of detail, such as a list of clinical conditions that a student should encounter and master during a course. There are several ways of doing this, the two most popular being a systems-based model (cardiovascular, neuroscience, infection and immunity, etc.) and a life-cycle model (childhood, adolescence, adulthood, aged care, etc.). Both systems- and life-cycle-based organisation involve a degree of integration of curriculum material, but the integration is generally across basic biomedical and social sciences. This is known as *horizontal* integration.

The next layer of organisation involves grouping curriculum material into domains or themes. These are really just conceptual groups of similar content material that are usually present throughout the curriculum, rather than at specific year levels. The traditional organisation has been into *knowledge, skills* and *attitudes*, the three commonest broad conceptual areas of a curriculum. Current education practice goes beyond this to express curriculum content more elaborately, in terms of conceptual themes, including the attributes required by competent professionals. Knowledge is regarded as having to be applied in practice, not 'simple' knowledge. Skills now include a wide range of commun-ication, examination, procedural and information management skills. Attitudes now include a wide range of personal and professional behaviours, including legal and ethical behaviours. Finally, educators now realise that the traditional individual patient care model is no longer sufficient, so there is often a domain/theme about community and population health issues. Hence current domains or themes often have more specific nomenclature, reflecting this broader and more precise view of the desired attributes of graduates. Individual curricula may have between three and seven domains or themes, depending on the choice of the curriculum planners. The capacity of domains/themes to span years of curricula content is known as *vertical* integration. Integration is discussed further below.

The domain/theme-based approach does, however, have limitations. For a start, they are not easily definable, stable sets of issues that can be taught or assessed independently. Domains often overlap. For example, communication skills can be within both a skills domain (communication with patients and peers) and a professional behaviour domain (teamwork in the workplace).

Hence a more contemporary way of looking at what to teach (and assess) in medical education is to add a third level of organisation to a curriculum, by considering the *roles* that medical practitioners play. Again, there are several ways of looking at these, but all have in common the concept that medical practitioners must master knowledge, skills and attitudes that are relevant to patient care (previously the sole or primary focus), the function of the healthcare system and their own personal care as a professional person. Issues relevant to each of these three areas are given in Box 7.1, which lists the headings of the CanMEDS description (*see* Further reading).

Box 7.1 The roles of medical practitioners (from CanMEDS – *see* Further reading)

- Medical expert
- Manager
- Teacher
- Collaborator
- Communicator
- Researcher
- Health advocate
- Professional

Many of these role issues are more relevant in postgraduate training and continuing professional development, but medical school curricula should include them so that students understand from the beginning of their education the nature of their future roles. They should have opportunities to learn, and should be assessed on how they fulfil the roles of a medical practitioner. This approach often provides the answer to such questions as 'why is it important to learn about . . .?'. Several topics that do not seem directly relevant to patient care – for example, the acquisition of teaching, advocacy and management skills – can be seen as relevant to future practice, and should be included even in undergraduate medical curricula, but at a level appropriate to the expectations of medical students and new graduates.

Defining learning objectives

Curriculum material that is selected from a wide range of potential content (the 'universe' of medical curricula, indicated by the large box in Figure 7.1) and organised into domains/themes needs to be translated into learning objectives for students to aim at. There should be learning objectives for the overall medical course – it is best to consider the expectations of a graduate, ideally linked to the expected roles of medical graduates – but also for each year, phase or block of the course, and even down to the level of each teaching session. These learning objectives must all be congruent and flow logically over the duration of the course. That is, learning objectives for earlier phases, years, blocks or subjects should be subsumed by following years, phases, blocks, etc., leading to the final set of learning objectives for the course for graduating students. These objectives should be specific, as this guides teaching and learning better, and measurable, as this assists with assessment and evaluation processes (*see* Chapter 8). Some examples of specific, measurable learning objectives are provided in Box 7.2.

Box 7.2 Examples of specific, measurable learning objectives

By the end of the course, students will be able to:
- assess a patient with a renal problem
- formulate an accurate list of provisional diagnoses for renal problems
- order and correctly interpret relevant clinical investigations
- communicate this information effectively to the patient, the family, peers and other health professionals.

By the end of a more junior year, students will:
- know the normal structure and function of the renal system
- be able to identify renal structures in plain radiograph, ultrasound and computed tomography (CT) images
- be able to describe the filtration of blood by the kidneys to remove waste products
- be able to examine the renal system in patients
- be able to describe the impact of the overuse of analgesics on renal function.

By the end of a more senior year, students will be able to:
- take an accurate patient history relevant to the renal system
- conduct an accurate clinical examination of a patient with a renal problem
- determine a list of probable diagnoses.

Please note that these attempt to cover more than one domain for a selected human body system. Can you work out which ones address which kind of domain?

Box 7.2 also demonstrates how learning objectives can evolve over time from more junior to more senior years, phases or blocks of a curriculum. Those for the end of a course reflect a requirement for mastery of knowledge and clinical skills relevant to being a first-year medical graduate. In the more senior years, learning objectives reflect component knowledge and skills focused on pathology, whereas those in more junior years reflect mastery of components related to normal structure and function, plus some pathology. This hierarchy of learning objectives helps to define the depth of learning required at each level for the overall topic (e.g. renal medicine). Students feel much more comfortable when these kinds of depth indicators are available to guide their learning.

Curriculum blueprinting

This step is often omitted, but is a valuable implementation, assessment and evaluation tool. A *curriculum blueprint* is a way of making sure that the curriculum is implemented as it was intended and as it relates to healthcare. It begins with the structure of the curriculum, organised by (say) systems and domains, and then other relevant information is added to guide learning. Content is often better taught through problem cases, where the medical condition becomes a vehicle for learning. These medical conditions may be organised according to a recognised classification, such as the International Classification of Primary Care (ICPC), and are based on problems of attenders to primary care, or ICD-10, which is based on diagnoses in hospitals. Both are useful, depending on the learning objectives. Where possible, actual data on the incidence and presentation of the medical conditions should be used, as this approach is evidence-based. These data are generally available on a national and even regional level.

This information is often summarised in a curriculum blueprint, a very basic example of which is provided in Figure 7.2. Each box represents a component of competence that reflects a content area, here arranged by body system (a common approach) and domain of competence (row). In this example, only a single topic is provided for each content area, although clearly there are many that would be included in a genuine blueprint. Some domain-specific issues are relevant for more than the specified content topic, and would not necessarily need to be repeated for all conditions.

Figure 7.2 is a simple two-dimensional blueprint, and does not reflect the added complexity that exists in real life of medical conditions being found in people of all ages, both genders and several different ethnic groups. Where these issues are relevant, the information in Figure 7.2 can be further sorted to reflect those population characteristics, producing a three-dimensional blueprint.

Domains	Content area (International Classification of Primary Care)				
	Respiratory	Cardiovascular	Neurology	Gynaecology	Musculoskeletal
Knowledge	Wheeze and shortness of breath	Acute chest pain	Fits & faints	Abnormal vaginal bleeding	Painful joints
Clinical skills	Respiratory system examination	ECG: perform and interpret	CNS examination	Intimate genital examination	Joint examination skills
Doctor & community	Smoking, preventive management	Reducing cardiac risk factors	Identification, driving cars	Vaccination schedules	Rehabilitation
Ethical & professional	Should we treat asthmatics who smoke?	When to perform invasive investigations	Role of genetic screening	Arrangements for review	Overuse, syndromes and the workplace

Figure 7.2 An example of a simple medical curriculum blueprint.

A blueprint is more a conceptual framework than a precise definition, but can be a useful 'map' to guide curriculum implementation. In theory, learners should experience, and therefore potentially be assessed on, something in each of the blueprint squares. Course organisers can look at the whole blueprint and determine what should be taught by lectures, tutorials, workshops and practice-based supervision. Clinical teachers and learners can also inspect these documents and understand the relevance of their practice experiences to the broader picture.

Curriculum sequencing

A curriculum may be linear, in that learners progress through together at the same rate and in the same sequence, or it may be modular, in that discrete portions of the curriculum may be taken in varied sequences, often in a 'core plus options' model. The latter is the more common approach taken in higher education, as it allows the more self-directed approach that is preferred by adult learners. Medical schools often try to emulate this model, but often their curricula are so crowded that they are relatively linear, with only a limited range of options.

Curriculum integration

Curriculum integration is currently a popular concept. It means that curriculum components are linked in some way, usually with the aim of improving interest and relevance to learners. There are two broad kinds of integration. The first is *horizontal* integration, where subjects that could be taught in parallel are taught together. A common example is where anatomy, physiology and genetics are taught together, usually around an integrating theme such as human body systems – cardiovascular, respiratory, gastrointestinal, etc. The second kind is *vertical* integration, where subjects that are often taught in a linear sequence over several years are taught together, such as clinical and basic sciences, in a way that spans most or all years of the course. When clinical and basic sciences are taught together, the balance usually changes from the more junior stages (more basic than clinical) to more senior stages (more clinical than basic): this is often called an *overlapping wedge* model.

Domains/themes are often used as vertical integrators, as they include content in all years of a course and students are expected to develop the abilities over time. For example, clinical skills are now usually introduced early in a medical course at the same time as the medical science theory, again around an integrating theme such as body systems. These are built on each year, phase or block, until the endpoint learning objectives are achieved. Material may be visited in new contexts that are more elaborated in more senior years: this is often called a *spiral curriculum* model. Similarly, professional behaviour is expected to develop over time, based on teaching sessions and clinical experience in each year, phase or block of a course. Domains often form the basis of what are called *vertical streams*.

The spectrum of integration is wide, ranging from very little (almost tokenistic?) to high, where curriculum components are closely intertwined. Integrated curricula have two important consequences for medical schools. The first is that the higher the level of integration, the more complex becomes the organisation of the curriculum delivery. Whereas more linear and sequential curricula contain subjects that can be taught by a single teacher (or perhaps a small team), subjects in integrated curricula may involve many teachers who have to collaborate closely. The best way to explain this complexity is to develop *curriculum maps*, documents that demonstrate where and when in a curriculum the many components are taught. Curriculum maps come in many forms, by domains, subjects or disciplines, but should reflect the curriculum blueprint. Medical education units often devote considerable resources to developing curriculum maps as an aid to both implementation of the planned curriculum and helping particularly the part-time teaching staff to understand where their contribution fits in with the rest of the curriculum.

The other consequence of high levels of integration is that assessment is more complex, and again requires teams of assessors working together and assessing much more than just simple knowledge. Students find it more difficult to determine the depth of learning required and often become anxious about assessment. Few textbooks are written as integrated resources and most teachers have expertise in a relatively narrow range of subject or discipline areas, so a mismatch is likely between an integrated curriculum and the learning support systems. The most important method of learning in such a curriculum is to participate, so attendance becomes more important. Depth of learning is best guided through the use of well-designed integrated assessment methods and the provision of ample, timely formative assessment and feedback (*see* Chapter 8).

Implementing the correct curriculum

This at first may appear to be an odd heading, but the reality is that students can be faced with several different curricula at the same time. These reflect differences in the way a curriculum can be implemented, and are summarised in Box 7.3.

The *potential curriculum* is that which reflects all of the possible content that curriculum planners could think of, not necessarily to be a 'superdoc', but even just to become a basic medical graduate. Even at that level, it is not possible to formally teach everything that might be useful to be a basic medical graduate, and curriculum planners of all medical school curricula almost certainly debated hotly what was to be included in the valuable time and resource allocation for the contribution of each discipline. The strongest debate is often about what to leave out.

Box 7.3 Different kinds of curricula

- The potential curriculum
- The planned curriculum
- The delivered curriculum
- The assessed curriculum
- The hidden curriculum

The *planned curriculum* is, as it sounds, what the curriculum planners have agreed, after all that debate, will be included in the curriculum. This will often be very detailed, including domain maps, long lists of learning objectives and blueprints. As a result the curriculum may appear to be quite clear, with components of competence appearing to have precise relationships with each other. This is not often the way it is, but the simpler representation is a product of translating the detail into documents for curriculum implementers.

The conceptual difference between potential and planned curricula is illustrated in an oversimplified manner in Figure 7.3, which shows the relationship between a medical school curriculum, postgraduate curricula and the 'universe' of medical curriculum issues. The 'universe' of competence (i.e. everything that a pan-discipline medical genius might possibly know) is represented by the square, the planned medical school curriculum by the small inner circle, and the discipline-based curricula that span undergraduate and postgraduate education by the various shapes. The potential curriculum could include anything outside of the inner circle, perhaps dependent on the interests and understanding of individual clinical teachers who do not observe the boundaries of the planned curriculum. There are in fact more disciplines vying for a piece of the undergraduate curriculum pie than indicated in the figure; medical schools are frequently criticised for not meeting the expectations of, in particular, the newer, more specialised discipline groups.

The *delivered* curriculum is the delivery of the planned curriculum. This includes the lectures, seminars, practical sessions and clinical attachments that address the agreed learning objectives. The inherent obligation of all academic staff and clinical teachers is that they should be familiar with just what they are expected to help the students learn. This is particularly relevant for clinical teachers, who usually also teach postgraduate registrars and may find it easy to follow an approach that is more suited to postgraduate training in their specialty. At the undergraduate level, principles and concepts are often much more important than large amounts of factual information, although some of that is of course essential. Familiarity with curriculum maps and depth indicators are helpful here.

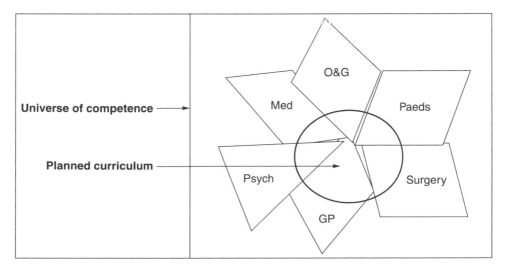

Figure 7.3 Relationship between a potential and planned curriculum.

The *assessed curriculum* reflects what students learn because they expect it will be assessed. Students are smart people who will not waste time learning what they think or know will not feature in examinations or other assessments, and will instead focus on what they perceive to be the 'real' curriculum. Assessment should therefore be based on the planned curriculum, as students who study that will be rewarded in the assessment process. This underlines the importance of assessing curriculum components such as ethical and professional behaviour, which are not easy to assess, but if they are not, students will not try to develop appropriately.

A *hidden curriculum* is what happens when the planned curriculum is not implemented as intended. This can occur for many reasons, including a mismatch between the planned, delivered and assessed curricula. This may be due to poor curriculum design, poor delivery or poor assessment practices. Was the planned curriculum realistic, achievable and supported by staff? Such problems may be prevented by placing the relatively complex process of curriculum design in the hands of people who understand medical education and change processes. Did well-intentioned teachers provide more depth than necessary in topics of personal interest or regarded personally as essential to the curriculum, even though that battle was lost in a curriculum planning meeting? Did these teachers role-model appropriate clinical and professional behaviour? Training clinical teachers (perhaps reading this book) should help minimise those kinds of problems. Did the recent curriculum focus on new content and delivery methods and simply adopt 'old' assessment methods, or (worse) was assessment developed independently of the curriculum? Again, assessment practices need to be designed by people with the necessary educational knowledge and skills.

An important message for clinical teachers is that they must realise that their students have to learn many things from many different people in different disciplines, ideally following the curriculum plan. Individual students may be inspired to exceed the requirements of particular disciplines at times, but they should not do this at the expense of required curriculum components. Wise clinical teachers realise that they are there for only a part of the student's journey, and take a broader view of helping students achieve the learning objectives of the curriculum now, and perhaps provide deeper discipline involvement at the postgraduate level. They should always role-model sound ethical and professional behaviour. If a clinical teacher demonstrates poor communication with patients or staff, when the curriculum talks about appropriate ethical and professional behaviour, which is the more potent shaper of young minds?

The relationship between the different kinds of curricula is presented conceptually in Figure 7.4. Ideally, the planned, delivered and assessed curricula should overlap entirely. When they do not, the result is confusion, with a 'hidden' curriculum emerging. This is what the learners experience, and comprises a combination of the other kinds of curricula in a way that may not be obvious to teachers and planners. If allowed to become the dominant driver of learning, a hidden curriculum has the potential to impede progress towards achievement of desired learning objectives. Clinical teachers have an important role in ensuring that formal curricula are both deliverable and delivered as intended, as the academics who develop curricula may not appreciate the practical issues of teaching and learning in clinical settings.

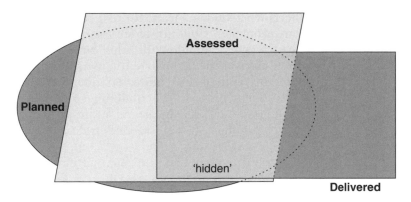

Figure 7.4 Curriculum 'wars': a conceptual diagram of how the 'hidden' curriculum develops.

Other kinds of curricula

Amidst the current wave of curriculum reforms clinical teachers will hear discussions about 'new', 'old', 'graduate entry', 'school-leaver entry', 'traditional', 'didactic', 'integrated', 'case-based' or 'problem-based' curricula. Evangelists exist for most possible curriculum formats and debates over which are the better can go on for years. Is any particular approach better than any other? This is not an easy question to answer, but to generate (or spark) controversy the following paragraph tries to do so.

Evidence from following up graduates of the pioneering problem-based learning (PBL) medical schools shows little difference in career choice outcomes, but that they enjoyed their learning more than students in the more traditional schools. Since then the question has become more or less irrelevant, as almost all schools throughout the world have adopted 'hybrid' approaches that include elements of didactic teaching, problem-based learning and early clinical exposure, all within integrated curriculum processes, and often also integrated assessment practices. Even the original PBL curricula have evolved, as their strength was in their early years rather than their clinical years and assessment processes. Few educationalists would argue against the value of PBL processes in encouraging a sound approach to problem solving, just as few would argue the need for students to learn a wide range of factual material as other tools, so long as they know they have to keep learning new and updated facts for the whole of their careers, or for sound assessment practices. The moral to the story is that the design and implementation of a curriculum is more important than any ideology behind particular curriculum methods.

The development of clinical reasoning

While some observers discuss medical courses as if they were linear, sequential competency-based programmes, universities believe that medical education is about much more than that. One example is that medical students are expected to develop clinical reasoning skills. I call this a skill for simplicity but it is less definable than, say, physical examination skills, but it is at the heart of how medical practitioners gather and synthesise information. It cannot be taught in a lecture, but can be *developed* in medical students, at least to a basic extent.

First, consider a bit of educational psychology theory. There are two ways in which doctors solve clinical problems. The first way is that we gather information, piece it together to form a hypothesis (or diagnosis) and then try to find information which confirms or refutes that hypothesis. This is called the hypothetico-deductive model of clinical reasoning. It is particularly useful for new, unusual or complex presentations. It may be used more often by internal medicine specialists than others, although there is not much proof for that statement. It can be slow, but is thorough. Not surprisingly, this is the way that learners start out in practice. Hence this method is used by both novices (for most cases) and experts (for complex cases).

However, it is not the way that experienced clinicians function most of the time. With experience, most presentations 'have been seen before'. Particularly when the doctor knows the patient, or has a semi-worked-up case referred from primary care, the patient's presenting complaint often fast-tracks thought processes to the point where a strong diagnostic impression is already present based on what might be called 'elaborated knowledge' and a library of patient scripts stored in memory. Fewer questions need to be asked to confirm this impression, so the whole process is over rapidly. This is called 'pattern matching'. It is used by generalists and specialists alike, perhaps more so by experienced narrower specialists who have simply seen a lot more of the unusual presentations than generalists. An analogy would be a CD-ROM with more images that can be accessed and matched more rapidly. At the extreme of the spectrum is the 'spot diagnosis'.

The difference between the two approaches comes down to experience. Pattern matching cannot be taught, but it can be learned. The most effective way of learning clinical problem solving is to encounter large numbers of clinical presentations. This is one rationale for presenting as much curriculum material as possible, including the 'basic' biomedical, behavioural and social sciences in early years, within clinical case scenarios. Ideally, these scenarios should be based on clinical presentations rather than diagnoses, replicating real clinical practice. During clinical placements an important role of clinical teachers is to ensure that their learners gain experience of several examples in each of a wide range of patient presentations. In time, the clinical clues fit into scored scripts in memory and a bigger picture appears sooner. The more clinical scripts are stored, the better.

There are two further forms of diagnostic reasoning that medical educators should try to prevent in their graduates. More recent research into how doctors gather information to solve clinical problems comes from the work of Page and Bordage (*see* Further reading). This work placed doctors into one of four categories: *reduced, dispersed, elaborate* and *compiled*. The last two correspond with, respectively, the hypothetico-deductive and the pattern-matching approaches of experienced, competent doctors. The first two probably indicate poor performance. Those in the *reduced* category just do not have enough knowledge to provide a basis on which to commence problem solving. Those in the *dispersed* category may have a lot of knowledge, but not the processing ability to rationally pursue information that helps make decisions. Instead, doctors in this second category seek exhaustive amounts of information, much of it not necessary to solve the clinical problem, and may well solve the problem (if they do) almost by accident.

The implications for clinical teaching are firstly that students should interact with as many patients as possible. Secondly, the experience of learners needs to be monitored to ensure a broad experience of clinical medicine. It is insufficient to assume that a suitable range of presentations will appear in any particular term, so students should be encouraged to seek opportunities in a wide range of clinical settings, including ambulatory and primary care, to interact with patients throughout the healthcare system. Third, clinical teachers should explain their diagnostic reasoning to their students, both as part of the role-modelling process and to explain to learners what they will observe in experienced clinicians. Learners are often amazed at just how quickly problems are solved, almost as if by some kind of 'magical' process that they cannot follow. They need to know that these leaps of intuition are indeed based on knowledge and experience, rather than luck. Fourth, while students may initially be encouraged to follow a more comprehensive approach to gathering clinical information, they should then be encouraged to look for patterns and associations that lead to a more focused approach, ideally one that is role-modelled by their clinical teachers. Finally, if clinical teachers recognise that students appear to have a *reduced* or *dispersed* approach, this should be reported to medical school staff as it may respond to remediation.

Although gaining a bigger store of memorised patient scripts is thought to improve diagnostic acumen, this is not an argument for learners to be pressured to see too many patients, too fast. There must be a balance between seeing and doing enough to increase the breadth of learning, and reflecting and discussing to add depth to the learning.

The relationship between the curriculum and clinical placements

This book does not attempt to provide a curriculum for clinical teaching, because that is provided by the relevant medical school. While much of a medical curriculum should probably occur in every medical course in the world, there will be local variations based on local healthcare issues. What the book does attempt to provide is a link between a curriculum, whatever its content, and the process of teaching and learning.

Many curricula are now accessible in interactive web-based formats, so the information required to be a medical graduate is easy to find. However, reading a curriculum, even discussing it with colleagues, does not provide the skills necessary to provide competent medical care. The power of clinical supervision lies in the ability of learners to apply their new knowledge in a healthcare setting, where patients and clinicians bring the curriculum to life. Clinical teaching is not so much about acquisition of knowledge (textbooks, lectures and tutorials provide that), but about developing clinical reasoning skills. This is best done by participating in a wide range of clinical encounters, observing and being observed by clinicians who know what to do. Participation includes practising talking to patients, examining them, formulating problem lists, working out what investigations to order and synthesising all that information towards making a management plan. This needs to be done with correct ethical and professional behaviour and by working as a member of the healthcare team. Role modelling of more senior colleagues is very important.

In some parts of the world medical students have relatively brief clinical placements and therefore rely on book learning in order to pass exams. These students sometimes seek long clinical electives in international healthcare systems, where they might put their knowledge into practice, sometimes without the benefit of close supervision. While the long-term outcomes may be similar, medical students who have the benefit of longer supervised clinical placements are probably more work-ready at graduation.

Summary

This chapter has provided an overview of current curriculum development issues in order to explain where clinical teaching fits into a broader curriculum framework. Some curriculum issues concepts have been summarised, and clinical teachers should read further on each of these issues should they wish to develop curriculum development expertise. Specific content issues are discussed where relevant to teaching and learning methods. The next chapter discusses the importance of assessment to clinical teaching.

Further reading

- CanMEDS 2000 (2000) Extract from the CanMEDS 2000 Project Societal Needs Working Group report. *Medical Teacher*. **22**: 549–54.
  This summaries the ground-breaking work from Canada that describes, perhaps better than others, the broader roles required of medical practitioners for current medical practice.
- Elstein AS, Schulman LS and Sprafka SA (1978) *Medical Problem Solving: an analysis of clinical reasoning*. Harvard University Press, Cambridge, MA.
  Almost the original seminal text explaining how doctors solve problems, but still worth reading for deeper understanding.
- General Medical Council (1997) *The New Doctor*. GMC, London.
- General Medical Council (2000) *Good Medical Practice*. GMC, London.
  Sequential publications that define for the UK what kind of medical practitioner is desired for the current time, and how to train those medical practitioners to be, and continue to be, sound practitioners. The principles are probably applicable elsewhere.
- Gordon J (2003) Fostering students' personal and professional development in medicine: a new framework for PPD. *Medical Education*. **37**: 341–9.
  A rationale for including a wide range of personal and professional issues in a modern medical curriculum.
- Harden RM and Davis M (1995) *The Core Curriculum with Options or Special Study*. AMEE Educational Module No. 5. Association of Medical Education in Europe, www.amee.org/, accessed October 2005.
  A simple explanation of the structure of the 'core plus options' curriculum model.
- Page G, Bordage G and Allen T (1995) Developing key-feature problems and examinations to assess clinical decision-making skills. *Academic Medicine*. **70**: 194–201.
  Contemporary theoretical explanations of clinical expertise and elaborated knowledge.

- Papadakis MA, Hodgson CS, Teherani A and Kohatsu ND (2004) Unprofessional behaviour in medical school is associated with subsequent disciplinary action by a state medical board. *Academic Medicine.* **79**: 244–9.
  Evidence that problem doctors were often problem students. Powerful evidence for including professional issues in teaching and assessment.
- Schmidt HG, Norman GR and Boshuizen HPA (1990) A cognitive theory on medical expertise: theory and implications. *Academic Medicine.* **65**: 611–21.
  A more recent explanation of clinical expertise and elaborated knowledge.

Chapter 8

Assessment and evaluation of learning in clinical settings

The craft so long [to learn], the life so short.
Hippocrates, 460–370 BC

Introduction

This chapter provides a brief overview of current theoretical issues in educational measurement applied for two purposes: assessment of individual student performance and evaluation of the teaching programme. These two purposes are quite distinct, but the underlying theory and terminology is quite similar, potentially leading to some confusion. Confusion can be exacerbated by reading the medical education research literature, as there are international variations in assessment terminology. In North America, student assessment is often known as student evaluation, so literature searches need to use both 'assessment' and 'evaluation' as key words when seeking information on student assessment, and then to decide whether the information is relevant to student assessment or to programme evaluation.

The chapter begins by explaining the inter-relationship between assessment and evaluation. For the rest of the chapter, assessment and evaluation are sometimes presented separately, indicating the differences between them, although wherever possible the characteristics and methods common to both their similarities are presented together. The provision of a deeper level of theory than that in Part 2 is intended to guide clinical teachers who want to explore the principles and issues that underpin assessment and evaluation practices, some of which are described in Chapters 5 and 6. Clinical teachers who join assessment or evaluation committees in medical schools or postgraduate certification organisations are likely to need this deeper understanding.

The relationship between teaching, assessing and evaluating

While it is easy to think of curriculum design, teaching, assessment and evaluation as separate issues, in reality they are closely inter-related. Figure 8.1 attempts to show this; note that this is very similar to Figure 7.1, but includes some additional arrows. There is now an arrow from assessment objectives to the curriculum content. Further, all arrows are two-way.

The curriculum, teaching and assessment components were covered in Chapter 7, so this section will focus on how evaluation fits in. The answer is that it can, and probably should, fit in at every stage. Evaluation can focus on to what extent the 'what should be known' reflects curriculum objectives and 'all that is known'; that might be of particular interest to funders and the broader community and professional groups. Evaluation can also focus on curriculum delivery (of interest to trainers of the teachers) or on assessment practices (of interest to university lawyers). Each level has an important role in the quality of a teaching programme and all levels should be considered in any comprehensive programme evaluation process.

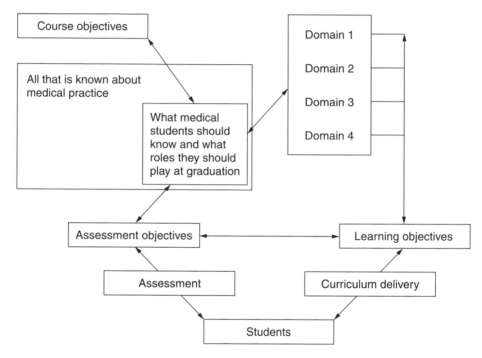

Figure 8.1 Curriculum structure and component relationships.

Assessing the roles of medical practitioners

It is worth highlighting that assessment must also reinforce learning about the currently expected roles that medical practitioners must play in professional practice. One of the landmark papers of recent years is the evidence that medical graduates appearing before the California Medical Board had a much higher chance of having documented behaviour problems in medical school than the rest of their cohorts (*see* Further reading). Medical boards have long suspected that this was the case, based on anecdotal evidence. Now that there is firmer evidence that problem behaviours in medical school might predict later problem behaviours in professional life, medical boards are very keen for medical schools to assess personal and professional behaviours and to intervene early. Clearly, clinical tutors have a responsibility to contribute to this process.

This, however, raises several difficult issues. What is the impact of maturity on professional behaviour? Many medical students are young, and probably not fully mature adults (students might disagree!). Is there a place for 'high spirits' and 'fooling around' in medical student behaviour? Should we be forgiving of students who behave 'stupidly', and let them off with a warning? How strong a predictor of future concerning behaviour is poor behaviour as a student? How can such behaviours be measured?

There are no easy answers to these questions, but the broader community currently expects high standards of the medical profession, including its more junior members. Each medical school will have clear guidelines about what are problem behaviours and what to do about them. It is best to focus on known problem behaviours – for example, breaching confidentiality, disrespect for patients and colleagues, poor attendance, alcohol or drug dependency – particularly if these are repeated and become persistent. Perhaps everybody can be forgiven occasional, single lapses – but they must still be recorded – and the most significant predictor of future problems may be an unwillingness or inability to learn from experience and improve behaviour.

What is assessment?

Assessment could be defined as the measurement of achievement of progress towards meeting defined educational objectives. There are several different kinds of assessment, each with a different purpose, and clinical teachers are likely to encounter all of them. These are formative assessment, summative assessment and programme evaluation. A fourth variant is in-training assessment, which could be viewed as a hybrid of formative and summative assessment. The purpose of the assessment should always be clear to all participants.

Formative assessment

Formative assessment is that which provides feedback to learners in order to guide progress. Individuals learn in different ways and at different rates, and formative assessment offers opportunities for self-paced assessment of progress towards goals. Learners can be open about their strengths and weaknesses and seek advice from their teachers, agreeing on what might be done to address recognised weaknesses to achieve 'mastery' of learning objectives. Formative assessment is an essential part of any good educational programme. When performed correctly, few learners should be troubled by assessments at the end of a course.

On the other hand, formative assessment can be so individualised, time-consuming and almost *ad hoc* that it does not easily lead to a clear decision that all learners have achieved all necessary learning objectives at a given point in time. Indeed, by definition formative assessment should never be used to make a decision about an individual learner's progress. No medical school is quite confident enough in formative assessment practices to rely completely on it, although a couple of medical schools have experimented rather controversially with assessment programmes with either no, or a very small, final examination hurdle.

Summative assessment

Summative assessment is that which indicates that a particular level of competence has been achieved at the end of either part, or all, of the course. This usually means big (at least emotionally) examinations that inform decisions about the suitability of individuals to proceed to the next year or to exit a course with a degree or diploma. This decision-making role of summative assessment is responsible for the unpopularity of examinations – nobody wants to fail and examiners do not like failing their students. Please note that such decisions do not necessarily mean that individuals who have passed summative assessment will always provide high-quality medical services, but rather that at a particular time the individuals were able to demonstrate the necessary knowledge and skills.

Apart from demonstrating that students are 'safe' to proceed, summative assessment has two very positive educational attributes. The first is that it can also have a formative role, as results can provide useful feedback to learners, whether they fail and must take a supplementary examination, or pass and know what they must work on to improve at the next stage. Second, well-designed summative assessment that is matched to course objectives and uses appropriate assessment methods should fail only those with significant deficiencies.

In-training assessment

This is a form of assessment programme that combines formative and summative assessment into a continuous or progressive assessment programme. This addresses some of the weaknesses of end-point summative assessment, which tends to assess only a small sample of the necessary knowledge, skills and attitudes, generally on only a single occasion, and does it in contrived circumstances (e.g. an examination centre), not in the context of real patient care. Hence there is some logic in assessing some attributes summatively during training and closer to where they have to be applied in the real world of healthcare. Ethical and professional issues are often better assessed during courses (e.g. dress and behaviour codes, attendance), and clinical skills can be assessed with real patients more easily during clinical placements.

The principle is that learners have several opportunities, most of which are formative, but some of which are known to be summative. Learners should be aware of the purpose of any assessments conducted during training, summative measures should be based on actual performance in the practice setting, feedback should still be given, and a flexible approach should be taken to timing and sequencing of summative assessments. In-training assessment (ITA) is discussed in more detail elsewhere (*see* Further reading).

Balancing assessment

Assessment is a common source of stress for students, and sound assessment practices can reduce student stress. There are two relevant issues here. The first is the overall amount of assessment. One of the commonest errors made in medical education is to over-assess, particularly in summative mode. This is a particular problem in newer, more integrated curricula, where the front end of the curriculum might change substantially, but assessment processes continue from the former, less integrated curriculum. Teachers often wrongly believe that integrated curricula must assess each individual component, rather than the bigger picture.

Instead, integrated curricula should have well-designed integrated assessment methods that are matched to the curriculum process.

The second issue is the balance of formative and summative assessment. Formative assessment is an essential part of the learning process, is generally welcomed by learners, and should be frequent. On the other hand, summative assessment is about ensuring that learning objectives at certain stages have been achieved, and that learners are ready to move on to the next stage. It is less popular with students and is more stressful. However, well-designed summative assessment does not have to be overly time-consuming. Formative assessment should therefore substantially outweigh summative assessment.

What is evaluation?

By definition, evaluation is *measurement against a standard, for a purpose.* If only it were this easy! The reason why evaluation is not easy is that it is uncommon to have a precise standard against which to measure. In educational evaluation, the stated educational objectives of the teaching programme are often used as standards, which are often called *benchmarks*.

Programme evaluation is a broad term that includes a wide range of measurement activities that can indicate how well a course is meeting educational objectives. Medical schools should conduct regular evaluations of teaching performance as part of programme evaluation, and this information should be openly available to all teaching staff. An example of why it is important was given in Chapter 6; course organisers often blame unexpectedly poor assessment results on the learners ('a bad group'), when it is more likely that either the curriculum implementation or the assessment was inappropriate. Programme evaluation is the means of working out why things turned out as they did.

As with assessment, evaluation can be either formative or summative, although these terms are used less frequently. Instead, evaluation designed to guide improvement is often called *developmental* evaluation or *quality improvement.* Where decisions are made about programmes on the basis of an evaluation, the process is usually called *accreditation.* The purpose should always be clear to all participants, as behaviour can change if participants fear a negative outcome (e.g. loss of funding for a project).

Continuous quality improvement

Most evaluation processes are regarded as quality improvement and should be regarded as a continuous cycle of activities, as is summarised in Figure 8.2. Please note that this cycle is evident in Figure 8.1, although in a more complex way. The philosophy should be that all teaching and all teachers can improve, similar to that which underpins clinical quality assurance programmes. A programme will include objectives, which are implemented. At some point activity is measured against the original objectives, and the results are interpreted as showing progress towards meeting the original objectives. This measure, which may exceed the original objectives, then defines a new internal benchmark against which activity will again be measured, and so on. The strengths of this continuous quality improvement (CQI) model is that wherever a programme is found to be in relation to the starting point, the idea is to move on and improve against internal benchmarks. A weakness is that it can be difficult to use external benchmarks (not many are available) and so comparing programmes in these processes can be difficult. The degree of active participation in such evaluation is probably the most important measure sought by external organisations.

Accreditation

In concept accreditation is similar to in-training assessment, in that a combination of measures can be used, with a combination of internal and external benchmarks, and a combination of quality improvement and decision making. Medical schools are familiar with accreditation processes as they are a common means of maintaining standards of medical education within national jurisdictions. More recently, the World Federation of Medical Education has developed international standards for medical education, although these are designed for a CQI model rather than decision making.

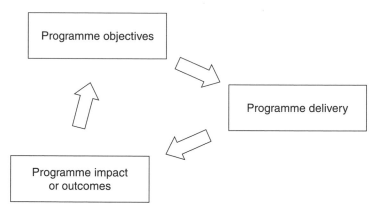

Figure 8.2 The CQI cycle.

Characteristics of sound assessment and evaluation practices

Both assessment and evaluation involve measurement of information, both quantitative and qualitative. In assessment, the focus of the measurement is the student, whereas in evaluation the focus is the curriculum. Before discussing individual methods, the characteristics of sound measurement practices should be considered. While there may be no such thing as 'perfect' assessment or evaluation practices, sound practices should reflect the six characteristics listed in Box 8.1. All forms of assessment and evaluation measurement display these characteristics to a greater or lesser extent, and all are important. Sadly, much debate on assessment practices focuses on the first two, when a balanced approach to assessment should include consideration of all six.

The first characteristic is *validity,* or the capacity to assess that which is intended to be assessed. There are several kinds of validity, as listed in the glossary of terms (*see* p. 150), but all relate to measuring the correct attributes. Ideally, they relate to learning objectives of the particular course, which in turn reflect community and professional expectations.

Box 8.1 Attributes of assessment and evaluation measurement practices

- Validity
- Reliability
- Educational impact
- Acceptability
- Feasibility
- Efficiency

The second characteristic is *reliability*, or the capacity to produce the same result if the measurement is repeated. This is important because a medical course should neither pass those who do not know enough for safe practice, nor fail those who do know enough for safe practice. Increasingly, students who fail consider appealing the decision and even taking formal legal action, so medical education units devote resources to measuring reliability (an evaluation measure for assessment) to ensure pass/fail decisions are defensible. Some educationalists worry about the potential for conflict between validity and reliability. In theory, validity and reliability should both be high, but in practice, many assessment methods regarded as having high validity demonstrate poor reliability. This is not, as some argue, because validity and reliability are opposing ends of the assessment spectrum, but rather because medical education research has not yet developed reliable methods of assessing some of those attributes now regarded as essential for medical practice. However, while it is true to say that there is a tension between validity and reliability across the assessment spectrum, both are important.

The third characteristic is the *impact on the learning process* of students or the curriculum. Most will have heard the truism that 'assessment drives learning'. This is usually cited as a criticism of assessment, but good assessment practices use this characteristic in a positive way, by employing assessment methods that measure the intended attributes (validity), and therefore reinforce intended learning. Evaluation can determine how well the assessed curriculum matches the planned and delivered curricula.

The fourth is the *acceptability* of the assessment. This includes a range of community and professional ethical considerations that might have different emphases in certain contexts. For example, using covert standardised patients is a powerful method of performance assessment that is acceptable in some countries, but not in others. Similarly, is it acceptable to use covert 'simulated students' to evaluate teaching and assessment practices?

The fifth is *feasibility*, or the capacity for the assessment and evaluation practices to consume resources, such as time, money and personnel. Many measurement practices are criticised because they are highly resource-intensive, but in reality most assessment methods occupy a great deal of time, space and other resources. In general, resource issues should not impede development of improved assessment and evaluation practices, as it is likely that use of resources will simply change, rather than increase. High-cost evaluation processes are harder to justify as evaluation budgets are generally quite small.

The sixth is *efficiency*, a psychometric property that for assessment practices indicates the capacity to produce an acceptable result with optimal use of examiners, test cases and particular test formats. The evaluation of assessment methods requires particular psychometric approaches that are not dealt with in any detail by this book. For evaluation practices, the concept is similar, but as yet there does not appear to be an equivalent measurement of efficiency. Here, the concept probably includes the issues of efficient collection of evaluation information (ideally built into implementation processes, or *evaluation by design*), and timeliness, which relates to how soon evaluation results are available to influence future implementation.

In student assessment, these attributes are conceptually combined to form a *utility index*. This is a useful concept as it demonstrates that reliability and validity are not always the most important attributes of assessment in the real world. A more detailed discussion of these attributes of assessment is suggested in the Further reading list (Van der Vleuten, 1996). This term is not applied to evaluation practice, although the parallel concept is present.

Setting the standard

For all measurements that require some kind of decision, there needs to be some information with which to compare the measurement. In student assessment this is called the standard, in programme evaluation it is often called a benchmark, although the term 'gold standard' is used for that somewhat mythical ideal situation that is probably not achievable.

Discussions about standard setting can be confusing because there is no ideal way, and certainly no single way, to determine a particular standard against which to compare. Amidst this uncertainty many different methods are used to determine a standard score. Benchmarking in some aspects of evaluation is more complex than standard setting in student assessment, because the approach requires a combination of quantitative and qualitative information, and the quantitative information reflects smaller numbers and therefore less useful statistics. Ultimately, setting standards requires judgements by people, but there are ways of improving the precision and acceptability of the standards.

Setting standards for student assessment

In student assessment, medical students tend to be academically bright high achievers and many clinical teachers, who themselves always performed well, have high expectations of their students. Some clinical teachers enjoy helping students to develop very high levels of achievement in their own specialty area, and indeed it is possible for a medical student to be as knowledgeable as a registrar about some clinical topics. At the opposite end of the spectrum there may be a few students who are struggling, more likely for personal than academic reasons. Clinical teachers may get to know these students very well and might feel inclined to be forgiving should they not meet the expected standards.

Neither situation reflects what medical school curricula aim to achieve. Medical students are expected to achieve defined learning objectives across a wide range of clinical topics and disciplines, as indicated in the curriculum. Experienced assessors may have developed an intuitive understanding of what is an acceptable standard, but new assessors may need to think carefully through the issues in order to reach this point faster than their experience alone allows. Hence a brief explanation of how to set standards is worthwhile.

Individuals are assessed against some kind of standard, which is used to determine a pass/fail decision and, often, grades of passes. Two important questions are: what is the most appropriate standard and how is this determined for a given assessment?

Relative and absolute standards

The first issue is the method of determining the appropriate standard. There are two broad approaches: norm referencing and criterion referencing. Norm referencing is comparison against the peer group. An example of this is a high-jump competition, where the winner is the one who jumps highest on the day, no matter what that height is. In terms of an examination paper, norm referencing might set the pass mark at the score that excludes the bottom 10%. A 'distinction' could be awarded to candidates whose scores were in the top (say) 10% of scores. This means that decisions about grades and failing are made relative to the scores of all candidates at the particular examination, and that the proportion of failing candidates remains stable in all examinations. Another term for relative standards is norm-referenced standards. This approach is infrequently used in medical student assessment.

The alternative approach is to determine absolute standards for passing and grades that reflect what students should know. With this criterion-referencing approach, the pass rates may vary between examinations, reflecting the reality that all examination cohorts are unlikely to contain equal proportions of very bright or poor students. To return to the example of the high-jump competition, judges could determine that the gold medal would be awarded only if a height of 2.5 metres is achieved. Should no competitor achieve this, then no gold medal would be awarded. Alternatively, should two manage to clear this height, then two gold medals would be awarded. In terms of sporting competitions, this approach seems odd!

A common compromise in assessment is to set the pass mark at 50% of the total score. This means that a different proportion of students can fail each time, depending on their abilities. Some examiners would argue that 50% is too low, and set the passing score at 60% or 70%, or perhaps even higher. This is an absolute standard, but falls into the trap of not recognising that the 'real' pass mark should perhaps be 47% or 63%, and will probably vary between examinations. This is not a truly criterion-referenced method, as it does not consider the degree of difficulty of the assessment process. The lack of precision around the pass mark also highlights the difficulty presented by students with scores near the passing score; should they pass or fail?

Dealing with borderline scores

In medical education the most significant issue is not really how to deal with either the clearly high achievers (they will keep going and probably do well) or the clearly low achievers (they need to do more work before proceeding). Wherever the pass mark is, is a student with a 1% higher score 'safe' to proceed and is one with a 1% lower score 'unsafe' to proceed? What about 2%, or 5%, either way? It is likely that a few students are awarded a fail when they should pass, and that a few are awarded a pass when they should fail. This is a critical issue in high-stakes assessment, where the emphasis should probably be on ensuring that only the 'safe' proceed to practice.

A common approach is to define a borderline zone within one or two standard deviations below the mean score. While this method is rational, in that it recognises the lack of precision inherent in scores, it is a norm-referenced approach, relating scores of individuals to those of the whole cohort.

Medical courses have escaped unwanted attention on the imprecision of passing scores because most students are academically bright and so the bell-curve is skewed strongly towards the right. Therefore almost all students are destined to pass and results can be ranked to identify the honours students. However, this is no longer acceptable, as allowing a poor student to graduate is potentially dangerous. Further, students who 'fail' are increasingly likely to take legal action, and having sound standards is a useful defence.

In medical student assessment there are two priorities. First, it is probably more important to ensure that all learners have achieved a particular level of competence than to award gold medals. This is why many medical schools have adopted non-graded pass/fail assessment decision-making processes for most of the course, even if they find a way to award a grade point average (GPA) or some similar ranking by graduation. This approach in theory encourages students to collaborate in their learning, discouraging the intense competition that sometimes results in textbooks disappearing or having key pages ripped out, but many medical students need the feedback that they are excelling to maintain motivation to do well. The second priority is that it is essential to define as clearly as possible the cut-off score between passing and failing scores.

Better definition of cut-off scores is inherent in criterion referencing, although most so-called absolute standards include an element of relativity to the performance of others; in the absence of an ideal method, pragmatism must prevail. Developing criterion-referenced assessment is hard work, as it requires test developers to carefully consider how candidates should respond to the test items, either together or individually. One approach requires a panel of clinicians to moderate each assessment item and determine just what constitutes a *minimum pass level* (MPL) for each item. There are many methods to choose from (*see* Further reading), and the application is probably more important than the particular method chosen. Further, a better statistical tool in determining cut-offs is to use the *Standard Error of Measurement* (S_E, sometimes confusingly labelled as SEM), which more accurately measures the reliability of any score, not just the mean. The formula is as follows: $S_E = SD\sqrt{(1-r)}$, where r is a reliability coefficient (e.g. Cronbach's *alpha*).

Benchmarking for evaluation

This is at once both more complex and more simple. The complexity arises from the multiple potential issues that may be evaluated and the complexity of combining quantitative and qualitative information. The simplicity comes about because a more pragmatic approach is therefore taken. A common approach is to develop *consensus standards*, reflecting the judgements of a wide range of stakeholders who may have a legitimate and relevant view of what the benchmarks should be. These consensus benchmarks are often at two levels that reflect the CQI philosophy that is so prominent in educational evaluation. These are *basic* standards, which attempt to define the least that is desirable for the present time, and *quality development* standards, which attempt to define higher standards to which an educational programme might aspire. The former could be regarded as the equivalent of norm referencing, and the latter the equivalent of criterion referencing.

Sets of standards for evaluation usually comprise large documents that include standards that reflect desirable or essential attributes, evidence-based and measurable criteria for each standard, and indicators that guide the measurement of the standards. Evaluators are usually required to record their judgements (met or not met) and a description of any issues or problems. The CQI philosophy requires the organisation being evaluated to both compare itself, and be compared against, one or both sets of standards, and then be given the opportunity to improve prior to any re-evaluation. Generally the more powerful motivator for change is the self-evaluation, particularly if it is reinforced by the external evaluation.

Measurement hierarchies in assessment and evaluation

The nature of the measurement in both assessment and evaluation changes according to contextual information that shapes levels of assessment or evaluation.

Levels of assessment

Standard setting and calibration of assessors are influenced by the level of the assessment for several reasons. First, the expected standards of performance should be different for students in early years, as compared to those in more senior years of the course. This does not mean that the same clinical cases (written scenarios, simulated patients or real patients) cannot be used in assessment at different levels, but that the tasks and the standards expected should be different. Ideally, assessment items are specifically designed to match the expected level of achievement of the target group.

Second, consider how students at more advanced levels of the course use knowledge and skills, compared with students at less advanced levels. Curricula often claim to revisit core concepts and knowledge repeatedly through the years to reinforce knowledge in clinical contexts – the *spiral* curriculum concept – and assessing knowledge and skills from earlier years is quite acceptable, even desirable. However, this should be done through the clinical contexts encountered in the more advanced years. For example, understanding of acid-base balance can easily be assessed in the context of a seriously ill patient in an intensive care unit, rather than a basic mathematical equation that assesses understanding of basic concepts.

Third, consider whether the assessment intends to determine the competence or the performance of students. Competence reflects the level of what individuals can do under certain conditions, usually highly controlled simulated conditions. Competence is the most desirable level of assessment for students at the end of a course or for registrars at the end of specialty training, where a reliable and therefore defensible decision can be made about candidates prior to graduation or licensing. Performance reflects what individuals do in their regular work, and has a closer relationship with healthcare outcomes. This level of assessment is not commonly used in medical student assessment, as students are not formally part of the healthcare team and have little responsibility. However, performance assessment is ideal for the assessment of medical students' professional and ethical behaviour.

The relationship between competence and performance is complex. Competence is most likely subsumed by performance, as illustrated in Figure 8.3. It is difficult to imagine that an individual health practitioner could perform well without achieving competence, but the reverse is not necessarily true, as it is quite possible for an individual who has demonstrated competence at an examination to subsequently perform poorly. There may be a gap between what an individual knows what to do and what they actually do. This should not be surprising, as the two are quite different. Performance assessment is the most desirable for professionals practising in the community, as we are interested in what actually happens. The significance of this distinction is that different assessment methods may be required for each level, as is illustrated in Figure 8.4, an adaptation of 'Miller's pyramid' (*see* Further reading).

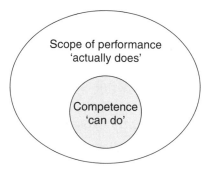

Figure 8.3 Relationship of competence to performance.

Fourth, consider how the assessment fits into professional hierarchies. Health professionals face several different levels of assessment, depending on their professional status. At the first level, as students, they are likely to be assessed on component knowledge and skills that, when combined, produce professional competence. At the end of their course, they take competency examinations, which assess fitness to enter professional preparation courses. This level is often called 'licensure', particularly if there is a national competency assessment. Following professional preparation courses, they take more integrated clinical examinations, which measure fitness to enter unsupervised professional practice. This level is often called 'certification'. Following a period of supervised professional practice, they undertake assessments that demonstrate continuing fitness to practise. This 'recertification' assessment should be performance-based. Finally, individuals with suspect poor performance may be required to undertake assessments, also performance-based, which are used to diagnose deficiencies in order to plan remediation programmes. This perspective on professional assessment indicates how high the stakes can be in assessment of health professionals, particularly at the upper end. It is important to develop the best possible assessment programme, so that decisions are as correct as possible.

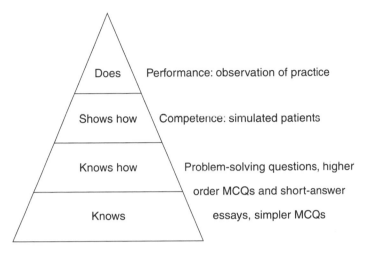

Figure 8.4 Modified Miller's pyramid (after Miller, 1990).

Levels of evaluation

Any teaching programme includes many different steps, processes and resources. Evaluation of a teaching programme can therefore be focused on any of these individual steps, processes or resources, or on various combinations of them, or on all together. There are several ways of looking at these.

Structure–process–impact–outcome evaluation

One useful way of looking at evaluation is to consider whether or not it is focused on the *structure* of the teaching programme (the 'what' – the curriculum content, resources, etc.), the *process* (the 'how' – scheduling, teaching methods, etc.), the *impact* (short-term effects or results) or the *outcomes* (long-term results). The outcomes generate the most interest, but can be the hardest to measure (e.g. death rates of the population as a measure of the success of medical education).

An eight-level hierarchy of evaluation measures designed for health education is summarised in Table 8.1. Clearly, level 7 is the ideal, but it is difficult to achieve. Level 4 is probably the most commonly achieved level of educational evaluation seen in medical schools. Going beyond this level with medical students is difficult and requires expertise that cannot easily be transferred by reading a small book like this. Advice should be available from the medical education unit in each medical school.

Individual–group–whole cohort evaluation

Structure, process, impact and outcome can all be measured from the perspective of individual learners, a small group of learners or a whole cohort of learners. A further stage is where a whole education programme is evaluated, such as during accreditation processes.

Table 8.1 A hierarchy of evaluation of teaching (after Pitts *et al.*, 1995)

Level	Description of measures
0	Nil
1	Satisfaction
2	Educational objectives listed and coverage
3	Wider educational needs sought and coverage
4	Learning outcome assessed – knowledge or skills
5	Learning outcome assessed – attitudes change
6	Learning outcome assessed – change in behaviour
7	Health benefit outcomes – improvement in patient care

Choosing what to assess

In neither student assessment nor programme evaluation is it possible to assess all activities within reasonable resource and time constraints. Hence only a limited range of measures is usually undertaken and these should be selected by a rational process. In student assessment the rational process involves blueprinting and sampling, while in evaluation a somewhat similar process is followed. The choice of measures is very important as it will influence both the validity of the process and the measurement methods selected.

Assessment blueprinting

To ensure that assessment reflects the curriculum, individual test items should reflect the components of competence in the curriculum blueprint, now called an assessment blueprint. Development of a curriculum blueprint was discussed in Chapter 7. In theory, test items could come from any or all of the squares in Figure 7.2. However, it is rarely feasible to assess something from every box in the blueprint, so test developers must sample components of competence for testing.

Sampling

There are usually time and resources for only a small proportion of components of competence to be assessed, so determining which to assess is an important issue. Ideally, sampling of test items from a bank of items is done randomly, as this removes one form of bias from the assessment. So long as the test item bank has a sufficient number of good items, then random selection should produce a fair assessment of the 'universe'. Random selection can be done within domains, in order to ensure that the assessment reflects a particular weighting of domains. For example, should ethical issues be required to comprise 20% of a course, then it should comprise 20% of all assessment. Similarly, applied knowledge might be required to be both 40% of the course and 40% of the assessment. Sometimes over-sampling is done to ensure that a particularly essential component of competence is weighted higher in assessment, but this should not be done often as it potentially distorts assessment and learning objectives. It is generally more important to sample as widely as possible from the 'components of competence', otherwise pass/fail decisions may be based on insufficient spread of the 'universe'.

A related issue is how to score items that assess 'critical' aspects of professional care. The temptation is to feel that 'if the candidate gets this question wrong, they should not be let loose on the public!' This concept is called the 'killer' question, a 'fatal flaw' or 'black-balling', and must be resisted. Instead, it has to be accepted that no professional gets every decision correct; there is an inbuilt error rate that cannot be corrected by examinations. There are two ways to deal with this issue at the level of medical students. The first is to assess 'essential' competencies prior to the formal examination, so that they become 'hurdles' to achieve prior to major assessment nodes. For example, it could be argued that CPR skills are essential for all health professionals, so all should be certified as competent in these as part of training (and frequently thereafter, throughout a career!). The second, and more difficult, is to ensure that the actual pass mark is criterion-referenced, through correct standard-setting procedures, as this should reduce the scope for making errors in judgements concerning what is 'safe' practice.

Integrated assessment

A further interesting issue is whether to assess individual curriculum components (subjects or domains) or the integration of those individual components. As a rule, the higher the level of the assessment (as in Table 8.1), the more appropriate it is to assess in an integrated manner. Newer curricula (both problem-based learning and hybrid) tend to teach and assess in an integrated manner from day one.

Particularly with professional practice, the most desirable method is to assess how individuals perform in the workplace. As professional practice requires integration of a range of domains of knowledge, skills and attitudes, it makes little sense to assess these individually. Professional practice is about dealing with real people and real problems, so the more the assessment focuses on these issues, the better. Writing integrated test items is not difficult, but requires teachers of particular parts of the course to accept that it is possible to assess their particular parts indirectly, as a building block of professional practice.

Evaluation mapping

Measurements for evaluation also need careful selection to ensure that the standards are measured. Standards documents provide information in an accessible format, with standards, criteria that together comprise the standards, and indicators that are measurable. Some standards are listed as *essential*, others as *desirable*. Much like an assessment blueprint, this information guides what and how to measure, with priority going to the essential criteria and standards. For medical schools, the relevant licensing authority for each jurisdiction (e.g. Australia and New Zealand, Europe or North America) generally has standards expected of their graduates. There is also a set of more generic international standards from the World Federation of Medical Education (*see* Further reading). These are very broad documents, including standards for most aspects of medical school function, and tend to focus on structure and process, but include sections on curriculum and assessment processes that are useful in thinking about how clinical teaching should be measured even in the absence of a formal review process.

Who should measure?

The traditional medical profession models have seen doctors assessing medical students and each other, because they know best, through intuitive understanding of the roles, what medical students and clinical teachers should do. However, this is a dated model and both assessment and evaluation judgements are now made by a wider range of people who are involved and can potentially make a contribution. Patients have a valuable role to play in student assessment, as they are the target of the students' endeavours. Similarly, students have a valuable role to play in programme evaluation, as they are the target of the education process. Self-assessment, peer assessment and expert assessment may have a role to play in most forms of assessment and evaluation. Note that in evaluation the term 'expert' here includes a wide range of people (nurses, other doctors from the same and different disciplines, patients, funders, healthcare and educational systems, etc.).

Patients (consumers of healthcare) are often in a better position to assess communication skills and humanitarian aspects of care, and now have a proven place in the assessment of general practitioners, and almost certainly can make a similar contribution in hospital and specialist care contexts. Similarly, the most valid assessments of teamwork skills and inter-professional communication can be made by nursing and other health staff who work with the students and medical staff in hospitals. Self-assessments are also valuable, mainly in formative assessment, as when compared to external (peer or supervisor) assessments they can increase self-awareness of performance in learners, an essential component of self-directed learning.

The situation is similar in programme evaluation. Doctors should no longer be the sole evaluator of a programme, and any doctors included should be external to the programme being evaluated. A more current approach sees a team of evaluators, perhaps four to eight individuals, each with a different background or area of expertise, and therefore different sets of expertise to apply to the evaluation tasks. For example: a community representative is ideal for exploring patient–doctor communication and access issues; a medical student is ideal in exploring the perceived value of teaching; and a representative of the funding organisation is ideal for exploring financial efficiency.

Of course the most important group to evaluate an educational programme is the staff and students of that same programme! In the CQI model, self-evaluation when done well discovers any issues that need addressing and motivates the staff to improve even before the evaluation report arrives. Understanding the programme is part of quality.

An overview of common assessment methods

The section on individual assessment methods is deliberately left to last because it is the last choice to be made in developing an assessment test. The correct sequence is to determine the curriculum content, including the learning objectives that now become assessment objectives. Next, select from the assessment blueprint the components that will be assessed, with allocation to domains and appropriate weighting. Third, standards should be set to guide the scorers of the assessments. Finally, the assessment method that is most appropriate for measuring the particular component is selected (*see* Further reading).

In most cases an assessment will comprise a combination of written and clinical tests, and will also likely include some assessments conducted during training, as these look at what the student is really doing. Both written and clinical assessment methods include a wide range of methods and these are summarised very briefly in Tables 8.2 and 8.3.

Table 8.2 Brief descriptions of commonly used written assessments

Written assessment method	Features
Essays	Assess written communication skills as well as knowledge/understanding. Lower reliability and efficiency as each essay takes a long time to write and mark.
Modified essay questions (MEQs)	Shorter than essays and can cover several issues at different stages; can be staged in steps; moderate reliability.
Short-answer questions (SAQs)	Shorter answers still; can cover several issues; moderate reliability.
Key-feature problems (KFPs)	Similar to SAQs but include clinical reasoning as well as knowledge; higher validity and reliability.
Problem-solving exercises (PSEs)	Like an essay with clinical reasoning built in by giving partial answers before asking next question; lower reliability and efficiency due to low numbers.
Multiple-choice questions (MCQs)	Many kinds but if well written have high validity, reliability and efficiency.
Extended matching questions (EMQs)	Provide so many choices that guessing is very difficult; higher validity and reliability.

It is important to realise that none of the methods included in Tables 8.2 and 8.3 are necessarily good or bad; all can play a role in assessment. Ideally, learners are exposed to several different assessment methods, as each one measures different attributes and a combination of methods is better than using only one or two methods at assessing a wide range of attributes or competencies.

Astute readers will note that Table 8.3 does not include Objective Structured Clinical Examinations (OSCEs), nor indeed the many variations on the theme (ISCEs, OSSEs, MSATs, etc.). This is because these are not really assessment methods, but rather assessment formats that include several different assessment methods. An OSCE is a combination of several, highly structured short clinical cases, and perhaps one or two longer cases, ideally all clinical simulations, and are now common in the more senior years of a medical course and beyond. The other variations on the theme include other assessment methods, such as laboratory tests, calculating drug doses, an evidence-based medicine exercise or even written task – potentially any discrete task that is a component of competence – and are most often found in earlier years of a course. A multi-station format of about three hours, including at least 12–16 stations, is likely to achieve defensible reliability while achieving reasonable validity, even though the clinical cases are not often genuine patients. Clinical teachers will almost certainly get involved with examining in OSCEs, where they will observe students with simulated or real patients and score them by completing a checklist, a rating scale, or both.

Table 8.3 Brief descriptions of commonly used clinical assessments

Clinical assessment method	Features
Short cases, a new version is mini-clinical examination (mini-CEX)	Replicate healthcare, so reasonable validity; if several included, reasonable reliability.
Long cases	Inefficient as use a lot of resources for assessment of single clinical case; hence reasonable validity but poor reliability.
Case studies	Combine written presentation with long case; similar attributes as long case and essays; high validity, reasonable reliability if several done.
Case presentations	Combine oral presentation with long case; reasonable validity but open to manipulation.
Viva	Open to manipulation by candidates; poor validity and reliability.

An overview of common evaluation methods

Evaluation practice requires a similar broad approach to that of student assessment. Evaluation requires a set of standards, criteria and indicators, a decision on which ones to select, and then election of the most appropriate measurement methods. While some methods include some measurement methods used in student assessment, evaluation usually includes a strong qualitative component. Common evaluation methods include content analysis of existing documentation, administration of questionnaires and conducting interviews. These are now discussed in more detail.

Analysis of existing information

It is likely that at least some evaluation questions can be answered through analysis of the material already collected about student learning and curriculum implementation. This may be recorded in a variety of instruments that record quantitative information, qualitative information, or both.

Just what is done with the information depends on the specific issue being evaluated and the nature of the information collected. At the level of structural evaluation, the question is the presence or absence of evidence that an appropriate teaching and learning environment exists. Teaching plans, teaching facilities, timetables, etc. provide the evidence, about which a judgement is made. For process evaluation, the question relates to how well this teaching and learning environment functioned. The frequency of particular educational strategies, the number of patients seen and practical procedures performed, how well course content was covered, etc. provide evidence for this. For impact evaluation, the question is what resulted from the teaching and learning environment. The results of formative and in-training assessments are relevant here, particularly if there are serial assessments that demonstrate change: self-assessments; peer assessments; patient assessments and supervisor assessments. The analysis of serial assessments can provide both numerical evidence of change (if there are numerical scales) or descriptions of performance and change. True outcome evaluation – how well learners later perform in practice – is not easily addressed at the level of clinical teaching, but requires sophisticated and complex data collection some years later when the graduates are in clinical practice.

Ideally, curriculum and assessment processes are designed and implemented with evaluation in mind. This provides the most efficient and timely evaluation, where data collection is infrequently duplicated and evaluation can be done as part of implementation, with results available for consideration, and perhaps implementation, very quickly. This *evaluation by design* principle is, however, rarely achieved amidst the pressures to deliver teaching and assessment with limited time and resources.

Should this ideal situation not be present, the use of existing data poses potentially strict constraints on its value in evaluation. Such data are often collected either for other reasons or in a manner that limits interpretation. For example, the most commonly recorded information is generally timetable information. It is necessary to inform students and staff about where they should be at what time. It can also indicate that a programme was provided and describe in general terms its content, but cannot provide any information on attendance or quality. Similarly, assessment results cannot provide direct information on teaching quality, as students will often prepare for examinations through strategies that are additional to (or omit) formal course requirements.

Questionnaires

An evaluation question might require information that is not available from existing sources. One method of collecting additional information is to ask learners to complete a questionnaire. This would be of value if the questionnaire concerns aspects of your teaching practice environment over a period of time, and involves several learners. In a sense, a questionnaire could be used to 'add together' perceptions of a series of learners or a series of patients. However, with small numbers of respondents, the ability to de-identify respondents is severely restricted, such that anonymity is difficult to attain. Hence, interpretation should be cautious.

Questionnaires are commonly used and often misused. A questionnaire is a highly structured method of gathering information. It has the advantage that it is easily administered, but the disadvantage that written words can be interpreted differently and clarification is not possible. These are potentially valuable sources of information, but are often designed and interpreted poorly. A poor questionnaire provides information that is either useless or irrelevant to the specific question in mind. Questionnaire design is a skill that few part-time evaluators will possess. Principles of questionnaire design include:

- careful selection of issues to be addressed. Avoid the temptation to ask more questions than are necessary.
- precise and concise wording to avoid ambiguity.
- careful layout to improve readability. Crowded questionnaires are more difficult to complete.
- a balance between types of questions. For example, ticking response boxes is easy for respondents, but provides less information. Free responses provide more information, but are more difficult to complete.
- piloting. All questionnaires should be completed by a small group of people to ensure that they are clear and unambiguous.
- sampling. Ideally, questionnaires should be sent to either a whole population of respondents (where numbers are small) or to a random sample of respondents. The former is the usual method for small numbers of learners.

Interpreting questionnaire-generated information also provides some traps for the unwary. Questionnaires produce opinions and perceptions of respondents; these are not necessarily correct, or even factual. High response rates within a target group can provide useful information that improves understanding of why individual respondents learned or behaved as they did, but they also mean that results are more likely to be applicable to the whole group. Also, questionnaires completed by learners in one practice will not necessarily reflect what is happening in another learning environment. However, questionnaires might provide information about the teaching and learning environment in a particular practice that is useful to the clinical supervisors in that practice. Those intending to use a questionnaire should seek advice from more experienced researchers.

Interviews

Interviewing learners, staff and patients about the teaching and learning environment can provide some rich information about a learning environment. An interviewer has the opportunity to respond to cues and explore these further. When conducted correctly, this method has the potential to provide the most valuable information about a teaching practice.

Interviews may be unstructured, semi-structured or tightly-structured. The former is the most difficult, but potentially most valuable, while the latter is easier but may not provide more information than a questionnaire. Interviews may also be of individuals, groups of similar individuals or groups of different categories of individuals. One of the best known forms of interview is a focus group. As an interview could be viewed as an 'oral' questionnaire, the above principles of questionnaire design are also applicable.

However, the traps are deeper here than for questionnaires. Designing an interview pro forma is as difficult as designing questions for a questionnaire. Interviewing requires skills in small group dynamics and an ability to monitor progress towards group objectives. The interpretation of information from interviews requires qualitative analysis skills. These are skills that few medical practitioners possess. The clinical teacher should probably not be the interviewer, the interpreter or the focus group facilitator, as he or she is one of the most important components of the teaching and learning environment and may find dispassionate objectivity difficult to achieve. Those interested in using interview methods should seek advice.

Summary

This chapter has presented further information on the more theoretical issues encountered in assessment and evaluation, and has provided a brief overview of those commonly employed in assessment and evaluation practices. Medical education units should be engaged in a constant cycle of developing curriculum and assessment practices that achieve a high utility index and maximise the likelihood of precise assessment that provides correct results. Similarly, all organisations should be in a continual cycle of monitoring and evaluating the entire teaching and assessment programme, to ensure that it meets the needs of the learners, the professions, the funders and the broader society.

Further reading

Evaluation

- Best JW and Kahn JV (1989) *Research in Education* (5e). Prentice-Hall, Englewood Cliffs, NJ.
  An overview of approaches to educational research and evaluation. Full of practical examples from classroom settings. Presents clear descriptions of how to create rating scales.
- Donabedian A (1988) The quality of care: how can it be assessed? *Journal of the American Medical Association.* 260: 1743–8.
  A clear explanation of the most often cited model of evaluation in healthcare.
- Pitts J, Percy D and Coles C (1995) Evaluating teaching. *Education for General Practice.* 6: 13–18.
  Describes a simple and meaningful hierarchy of evaluation in medical education.
- World Federation of Medical Education. *Quality Improvement in Basic Medical Education. WFME International Guidelines.* See: http://www.wfme.ku.dk/wfme
  Lists the WFME standards and reports on their use in international pilots.

Standard setting

- Cusimano MD (1996) Standard setting in medical education. *Academic Medicine.* 71 (Suppl.): S112–20.
  A comprehensive overview of current approaches to setting standards in assessment that explains complex methods in a practical, more reader-friendly way.
- Norcini JJ (2003) Setting standards on educational tests. *Medical Education.* 37: 464–9.
  One of the clearest explanations available for the theory and practice of standard settings.

Assessment

- Gordon J (2003) Assessing students' personal and professional development using portfolios and interviews. *Medical Education.* **37**: 335–40.
  Research showing that students rate positively the assessment of personal and professional development components in a medical curriculum.
- Greco M, Brownlea A and McGovern J (2001) Impact of feedback on the interpersonal skills of general practice registrars: results of a longitudinal study. *Medical Education.* **35**: 748–56.
  Research showing that patient feedback can help improve quality of interactions with doctors. The method has been used with medical students.
- Hays RB and Wellard R (1998) In-training assessment in postgraduate training for general practice. *Medical Education.* **35**: 307–12.
  This paper presents a conceptual framework for maintaining the roles of formative and summative assessment during postgraduate training, but the principles are probably equally relevant in undergraduate education.
- Joshi R, Ling F and Jaeger J (2004) Assessment of a 360 degree instrument to evaluate residents' competency in interpersonal and communication skills. *Academic Medicine.* **79**: 458–63.
  Research demonstrating that this method is reliable.
- Miller GE (1990) The assessment of clinical skills/competence/performance. *Academic Medicine.* **65** (Suppl.): S563–7.
  Describes the conceptual basis of competence and performance assessment.
- Newble D, Dauphinee D, Dawson-Saunders B *et al.* (1994) Guidelines for the development of effective and efficient procedures for the assessment of clinical competence. In: D Newble, B Jolly and R Wakeford (eds) *The Certification and Recertification of Doctors: issues in the assessment of clinical competence.* Cambridge University Press, Cambridge, pp. 69–91.
  Describes succinctly how to develop assessment processes, from beginning to end.
- Norcini JJ (2003) Peer assessment of competence. *Medical Education.* **37**: 539–43.
  Shows that peer assessment has to be used carefully if it is to be a meaningful contribution to decisions about student performance.
- Page G, Bordage G and Allen T (1995) Developing key-feature problems and examinations to assess clinical decision-making skills. *Academic Medicine.* **70**: 194–201.
  This describes the origin of the key-feature question format.
- Papadakis MA, Hodgson CS, Teherani A *et al.* (2004) Unprofessional behaviour in medical school is associated with subsequent disciplinary action by a state medical board. *Academic Medicine.* **79**: 244–9.
  Evidence that problem doctors were often problem students. Powerful evidence for including professional issues in teaching and assessment.
- Van der Vleuten CPM (1996) The assessment of professional competence: developments, research and practical implications. *Advances in Health Sciences Education.* **1**: 41–67.
  An authoritative view of the principles of assessment applied to health professionals, including a detailed explanation of the Utility Index concept.

A glossary of medical education terms

This appendix provides explanations of terms commonly used in educational and assessment circles. These are listed in alphabetical order, although some similar concepts are grouped.

Assessment is the measurement of particular attributes at a particular point in time.

> **Formative assessment** is assessment designed to inform learners about their progress towards achieving mastery of the course. In the context of the Royal Australian College of General Practitioners (RACGP) Training Programme, this means **feedback** and should be regarded as an integral part of teaching and learning. It includes observing, reviewing and informing learners about their progress towards mastering knowledge and skills.

> **In-training assessment** is the process of obtaining evidence in order to make judgements about the progress of learners towards attainment of the learning objectives of an educational programme. Methods used to collect such data include formal tests, assignments, projects, class presentations and reports. Evidence may be provided by self, peer or supervisors. Feedback should be given to learners for all in-training assessment.

> **Performance assessment** is the assessment of practice in the real world. It reflects what professionals actually do, rather than what they can do under examination conditions, which is **assessment of competence**.

> **Summative assessment** is assessment designed to make a decision about the suitability of a candidate to proceed to the next stage (e.g. from year 1 to year 2 or from learner to 'qualified'). The nature of summative assessment may vary according to how high the stakes are. For the RACGP Training Programme, the College examination is the summative assessment.

Checklist is an aid to structured scoring of answers. They vary from long detailed sub-components of desirable responses to more global categories.

Compensation of scores across subtests is the ability for strong performance in one subtest to make up for weak performance in another. This acknowledges that performance should be measured as a whole, rather than as scores of individual test methods.

Competencies are individual aspects of competence that can be learned and assessed.

Curriculum is a statement about the content of knowledge included in a training course and the process by which it will be learned. It is usually expressed in terms of learning objectives, domains and competencies. Ideally, a curriculum includes details of how learners will be assessed and how the training course will be evaluated.

Curriculum blueprint is a structured method of designing curriculum content, so that content reflects the learning objectives. Content is organised according to Domains or Themes, lists of common health problems or diagnoses, and age, gender and ethnicity.

Curriculum maps are a visual representation of the content of a curriculum component (Domain, Theme, Subject or Module) that ensures that the desired content is included and demonstrates relationships between individual topics. The result is a wide variety of complex diagrams.

Overlapping wedge describes a concept where the balance of basic and clinical curriculum content changes through a course. Initially there is more basic than clinical science; by the end this is reversed.

Spiral curriculum describes a concept where learners re-visit curriculum content repeatedly, each time at a different depth, with the aim of reinforcing its learning. This usually refers to basic medical, behavioural and social sciences, which may be covered early at a basic level, and then re-visited where relevant to clinical medicine.

Domains or areas of competence are conceptual groupings of competencies that organise and represent the main concepts incorporating the knowledge, skills and attitudes required for practice. Often also called **Themes**.

Error: assessment error is the term that acknowledges the inherent errors associated with any measurement.

Evaluation is measurement against a standard for a defined purpose. In education, this usually means measurement of the extent to which educational objectives have been achieved, and in the real world we must evaluate in situations where there are no definite standards. In the context of assessment, it means the collection of information to make a judgement about the reliability, validity, educational impact and efficiency of the assessment.

Hurdles are assessments that must be completed prior to taking summative assessment. These are ideal for assessing components of competence that are not easily measured by formal test methods.

Integration refers to the combination of different elements of a curriculum so that they are taught and assessed together in a way that links concepts, usually defined by body systems, life-cycle stages, Domains or Themes.

Horizontal integration describes the combined teaching across different subject areas. In medical education this usually means the teaching of anatomy, physiology and clinical material, etc., organised under body systems or life-cycle stages.

Vertical integration describes the linking of teaching content through areas of the course according to concepts that should develop throughout a course. In medical education this usually means the ability to apply knowledge and the development of skills and professional behaviours, etc., organised by Domains or Themes.

Learning objectives are clear, measurable statements about the expected educational outcomes of a training course.

Marking key is a structured 'ideal' answer to test items. It usually includes allocation of marks for parts of answers and should be prepared when the question or item is designed.

Objective Structured Clinical Examination (or Assessment) – OSCE (or OSCA) is an assessment format that combines several test methods, as appropriate for more integrated measurement of a range of competencies, particularly clinical and communication skills. It is not in itself a test method.

Psychometrics is the measurement of human behaviour and attributes. Complex methods are often used to achieve this. **Psychometricians** are those who practise the art.

Rating scale is an aid to structured scoring of answers, usually applied to clinical and communication skills assessments. There are two kinds: a semantic differential scale (very poor – poor – borderline – good – very good) and Likert scales (1–2–3–4–5). Different rating scales have unique measurement properties that need to be considered when combining scores of individual subtests.

> **Global rating scale** is a simple, often one-line scale that asks raters to assess overall performance. With experienced examiners, this is as reliable as more detailed methods.

Reliability of an assessment is the extent to which assessment results can be repeated on more than one occasion – the consistency of assessment.

> **Inter-rater reliability** concerns the consistency of measures by more than one observer.

> **Test–retest reliability** concerns the consistency of assessment scores when the same candidates face the same assessment on two or more occasions.

Reliability coefficients are a statistical method of producing a score between 0 and 1 that indicates the reliability of the assessment. In general, a score of 0.8 or more is regarded as acceptable. The most common reliability coefficients are **generalisability coefficients**, which allow sources of error to be identified as a guide to improving reliability.

Sampling of individual test items should be done randomly from an assessment blueprint. Random sampling works better with a larger bank of potential items. Stratified sampling is where items are sampled from within groupings with particular characteristics, such as domains, age groups, diagnoses, etc.

Standard Error of Measurement (SEM or S_E) is a statistical way of recognising both systematic and random error in measurement.

Standard setting is a process by which pass scores for each item and each test are determined on the basis of required level of performance, without reference to scores of candidates. Ideally, individual items have model, scored answers developed at the time of writing and agreed to by some sort of consensus process.

> **Norm-referenced (relative standard)** assessment: the performance of an individual is measured against the performance of the group as a whole. As

an example, a pass score may be set at 50% or by reference to mean scores for the group, rather than an external standard. Hence there tends to be a relatively fixed proportion of passes and failures.

Criterion-referenced (absolute standard) assessment: an external process that determines estimates of candidate performance and sets the passing score. As a result, the proportion of candidates passing may vary.

Test battery is a combination of more than one test method and/or format, or **subtests.**

Test blueprint is a structured method to guide sampling of individual test items. Wherever possible, this should reflect the universe of potential competencies and be based on data that defines those competencies, e.g. morbidity, age and gender data on presentations to general practice, domains of competence. *See* **Curriculum blueprint.**

Test format is an assessment mode e.g. written test, clinical test. There are several possible **test methods** within formats, such as MCQ and modified essay questions (written) and simulated patient encounter and observed physical examination (clinical). Each test method has strengths and weaknesses and may assess particular components better than others.

Themes. *See* Domains.

Triangulation is the measurement of an attribute, or group of attributes, from more than one perspective. Similar findings from different perspectives strengthen each other and the overall result.

Universe of competence includes all possible competencies in all domains. This may include attributes that are not easily assessed.

Validity of a test is the extent to which it measures what it is intended to measure.

> **Construct validity** is the extent to which assessment instruments measure the behaviours intended to be measured.
>
> **Content validity** is the extent to which a test measures the relevant clinical content.
>
> **Criterion validity** is the extent to which measurements agree with those of an accepted 'standard' test.
>
> **Face validity** is the extent to which a test appears to be acceptable to stakeholders.
>
> **Predictive validity** is the extent to which test performance predicts changes in behaviour (or other attributes) in the future.

Weighting of particular aspects of competence may be applied if there is evidence and agreement that these are more important than other aspects or components. Methods of weighting include over-sampling, awarding higher scores or creating hurdles.

Recommended resources for teaching units

Teaching units should of course provide access to a wide range of clinical resources to assist both clinical practice and learning. In addition, the following medical education resources can support the development of improved educational practice within clinical units.

Books

- Amin Z and Hoon Eng K (2003) *Basics in Medical Education*. World Scientific Publishing, Singapore.
  A useful primer for beginners in medical education.
- Newble D and Cannon R (1996) *A Handbook for Medical Teachers* (4e). Kluwer Academic Publishers, Dordrecht.
  Almost a classic, most useful for more formal teaching.
- Ramsden P (1996) *Learning to Teach in Higher Education*. Routledge, London.
  Provides greater theoretical and practical depth, but oriented towards more formal university teaching
- Robler MD, Edwards J and Havriluk MA (1997) *Integrating Educational Technology into Teaching*. Prentice-Hall, Englewood Cliffs, NJ.
  A bit techno-centric, but describes how to cross the interface quite well.

Journals

- *Academic Medicine*. American Association of Medical Colleges, Philadelphia.
  Strong research/methodology base, oriented towards North American contexts, but some useful articles, such as reviews of new books and educational software.
- *Medical Education*. Blackwell Science, Oxford.
  Strong research base. Includes reports on innovations, book reviews and short reports covering all aspects of medical education.
- *Medical Teacher*. Radcliffe Publishing, Oxford.
  More practical, wide range of topics, more relevant to UK and undergraduate contexts.
- *Teaching and Learning in Medicine*. Lawrence Erlbaum Associates, New York.
  Stronger research base, covering both undergraduate and postgraduate issues.

Most general medical journals also include occasional or regular contributions about teaching and learning issues:

- *British Medical Journal*
- *Canadian Medical Journal*

- *Journal of the American Medical Association*
- *Lancet*
- *Medical Journal of Australia*
- *New England Journal of Medicine.*

Websites

Net address (http://www.)	Theme
aamc.org	American Association of Medical Colleges
asme.org.uk	Association for the Study of Medical Education
bmj.com	*British Medical Journal*
blacksci.co.uk	The journal *Medical Education*
dundee.ac.uk/meded/amee	Association for Medical Education in Europe

Journal indexing databases

CINAHL – Citation Index for Nursing and Allied Health
Medline
SSCI – Social Sciences Citation Index. Often has educational research.

All medical schools have their own websites. Check on the address for the medical school with which you are affiliated.

Index